broken
heart

A nursing novella about coping with change and loss

Also by Amy Glenn Vega

LIONS AND TIGERS AND NURSES

Visit www.nursingnovellas.com
for exclusive information on titles
in the Amy Glenn Vega nursing novella series.

Available at www.p-h.com, or call 1-800-241-4925 to order.

amy glenn Vega

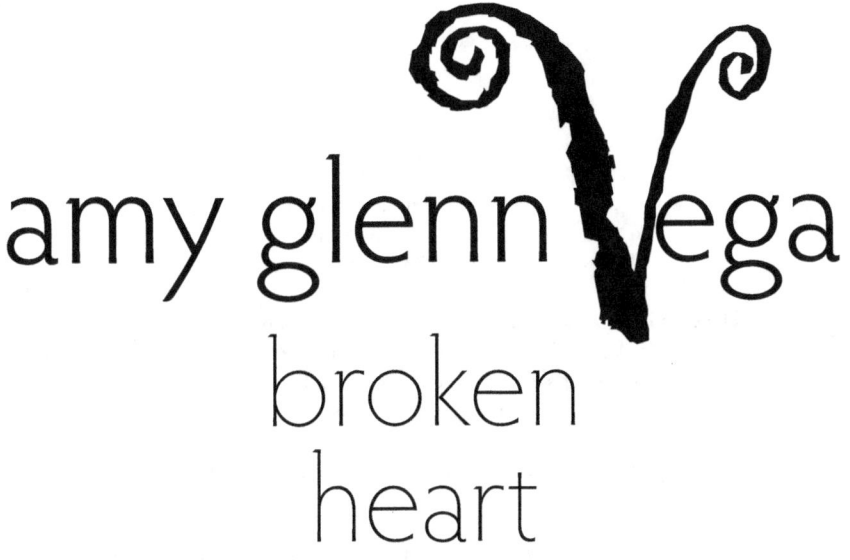

broken
heart

A nursing novella about coping with change and loss

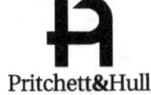

Pritchett&Hull

Published by
Pritchett & Hull Associates, Inc.
3440 Oakcliff Road, NE, Suite 126
Atlanta, GA 30340

For Frances

My grandma for the first thirty-three years of my life
And my guardian angel for all the rest
Thank you for loving me, for always being proud of me
And above all else, for showing me the difference
Between believing
And knowing.

ACKNOWLEDGMENTS

I suppose it shouldn't come as a shock that many of the acknowledgments for *Broken Heart*, a story that is largely about death and dying, would be for people who have already made that journey into the great unknown. But after reviewing my list of people to thank, I was pleasantly surprised by how deeply I continue to be influenced and inspired by the people who are gone from my life, but not from my heart.

I first and foremost want to acknowledge the work of the late Dr. Elisabeth Kübler-Ross, who dedicated her life to helping people throughout the world to understand death, and embrace it as a natural part of life. Her book *On Death and Dying* remains to this day a bestseller in the fields of Psychology and Thanatology. Today, the Elisabeth Kübler-Ross foundation continues her work. Its mission is "to build on the groundbreaking legacy of Elisabeth Kübler-Ross by confronting death and inspiring life."

I next owe a special thanks to Susan Parrish, MSN, RN, Director of the RN Residency Program at Cape Fear Valley Medical Center in Fayetteville, NC and David Carl, Director of Pastoral Care at Carolinas Medical Center in Charlotte, NC. The two of them kindly shared a wealth of information and real-world perspectives on how nurses cope with change, loss, death and dying.

Many thanks to the people who reviewed this story and provided the feedback that made it better. To my panel of nurse reviewers at Southern Regional AHEC, a special thanks to each of you: Jennifer Borton, Evelyn Clemmons, Sherri Eubanks, Andrea Novak, Saundra Stanley, and Deborah Teasley. Thanks also to Russet Hambrick for her thoughtful review of the first draft. A special thanks goes to my colleague and friend Karen Mantzouris, who reviewed this story alongside her sister, the late Alice Mazarick, RN, shortly before she passed away. With these words of thanks, I send out my prayers and wishes for peace to Alice, and trust that they will find their way to her.

Thank you Betty Westmoreland, Ken Baumann, Cecily Shull, Michael Austin, and the entire amazing team at Pritchett and Hull Associates, Inc. It is a joy and privilege to work with each of you and I take great pride in P&H being the publisher of this book. Our journey into the Nursing Novellas series has been delightful thus far, and I look forward to seeing which direction it will take us next!

Thank you again to my wonderful, supportive family and friends. I especially thank the late Frances Pridgen; my grandma, my other mother, and my friend, to whom this story is dedicated.

Thanks to a special family friend, the late Carole "Le" Longo, who would admire my early literary works written on the pages of my elementary school notebooks, and would tell me, "Amy, honey, don't you forget about me when you're rich and famous!" Le, to this day, I am still not rich nor famous, but now that I am a published author, I at least have the chance to let the whole world know that I have not forgotten you, and never will. Peace be with you, my friend.

Beverly Shelton, thank you for sharing your stories and words of wisdom about coping with the loss of patients in the Emergency Room, and how it has reminded you that life is a gift that should be lived to the fullest every single day. I hope that you will like your namesake character in this book and appreciate how she influences and inspires the nurses of Med-Surg South.

To my cousin, Heather Pridgen, thank you for sharing your real-world adventures of Med-Surg nursing with me. You are a great inspiration to this entire series.

Thank you once again to my mother, Karen Allen, for your never-ending support.

Thank you every nurse, in every corner of the world, both the living, and those who are living on through their legacy in nursing work.

And thank you, God, for nurses.

Dear Nurse,

Broken Heart is the second educational novella that I have written for nurses. Several people have asked me why I picked the topic of change and loss — largely, when it involves death and dying - to be the focus of one of the premier works in a series. The inspiration for this story can be traced back to a conversation a few years ago with my younger cousin, a new-to-practice nurse. "I lost a patient this week," she said to me, and the tone of our entire evening was from that point changed. She proceeded to tell me about how this post-op patient had bled out and gone into cardiac arrest, and how, in spite of the best efforts of an entire team of caregivers, they were unable to resuscitate him. She told me the patient's age. He was a young man, only a year or two older than she was. Death, of course, came unexpectedly for him. He had no will and no advanced directives. His physician was furious, and his family was devastated.

And behind her sad and troubled eyes, it was clear that my cousin's mind was working furiously to make sense of his death. After completing nursing school, she had chosen Medical/Surgical Nursing as her specialty area, with the very noble intention of helping people get well, go home, and get on with their lives. So what, she wondered, was this dying thing all about?

It's true; the thought of death and dying tends to make us all a bit uncomfortable. Most all of us have grieved the loss of family members and/or friends in our lifetime; all of us know that there will be more losses to come, and none of us have to be reminded of our own mortality. Death and dying may be the most universal topic that this educational series will ever touch upon. But for the nurse who is faced with death routinely, or even sporadically, there's more than just discomfort. There's the ever present danger of accumulated grief.

All nurses have had some training on death and dying at some point in their careers. If you need a refresher on the topic, the information isn't hard to come by. Look in any nursing textbook for information on the dying process or the grieving process, and you'll readily find it. A variety of national organizations and professional societies have developed wonderful, comprehensive curricula on end-of-life nursing care. The organization in which you are employed has its own policies and procedures, and no doubt, an interdisciplinary team of individuals at your disposal to help support the patient, the family and friends, and you - the nurse - through a patient's death.

The intent of this book is not to educate you with facts and statistics, nor arm you with clinical knowledge or skills for caring for your dying patient. Instead, this is a story that will allow you to explore the human side of death and dying. Through the eyes of five nurses, you'll share in their loss of two very different patients, and witness the different ways that they deal with it. You'll be reminded that losing a patient isn't just a loss for the loved ones; it's a loss for you too, and allowing yourself to grieve is normal, healthy, and healing. There's no one right way to grieve, but there is a common thread in healthy grieving, and it is finding and accessing a support system for as often and as long as it is needed. Loss can be difficult and painful, but doesn't have to be a burden that a person bears alone.

Before you turn the page, don't get the wrong idea about this story. It won't be all about death and dying. Like life itself, this story is a journey. With a beginning, an ending and some funny and exciting moments along the way. And as grieving is all about healing, so will the characters find some peace and resolution after the hard times. My hope is that in reading it, you'll be able to relate to some of these experiences, and draw some wisdom from them for when those difficult days come for you.

I applaud you for the good work that you do, and for the way that you make a difference in the lives of your patients and their loved ones. I hope this story will remind you that while you may not always have the cure for what ails your patients, you are always a healer.

Sincerely,

Amy Glenn Vega

"There is no joy without hardship. If not for death, would we appreciate life? If not for hate, would we know the ultimate goal is love? … At these moments you can either hold on to negativity and look for blame, or you can choose to heal and keep on loving."

Dr. Elisabeth Kübler-Ross

EDUCATIONAL OBJECTIVES

Upon completion of this educational activity, the learner should be able to:

1) Explain why every change is also a loss
2) Discuss the nurse's need to grieve the loss of a patient
3) Discuss how grieving behaviors differ between male and female nurses
4) Describe how nurses can support the patient, the family and loved ones, and each other when preparing for or recovering from a patient's death

Chapter 1
Monday
Mel

"Mom... I'm pregnant."

Mel Tagaro swallowed her last bite of vegetable egg roll and waited for the punchline. She forced a smile. "And?" She prompted Jenny, her nineteen-year old daughter, who was a sophomore at Western Carolina University with a 3.9 Grade Point Average and an indisputably bright future ahead of her.

Jenny stared back at her from across the tiny table and wondered to herself why she had chosen the Dogwood Town Centre Mall food court as the best place to break the news to her mother. "That's it. I'm pregnant. That's what I wanted to tell you."

Mel's smile faded. "You're joking, right?"

Jenny's lack of a response told Mel everything she needed to know.

"Oh my God. Jenny... what... who's the... I mean HOW? How could you let this happen?" Her eyes began to shimmer as tears formed.

Wringing her hands nervously, Jenny reached into her purse and pulled out a travel-size pack of tissues. "I knew you'd be upset, so I came prepared." She slid it across the table to her mother.

Mel sniffled and sat quietly for a moment, gathering her thoughts. "What are you going to do?" She finally asked.

Jenny took a deep breath. "I guess I'm going to have a baby," she replied.

Reaching for a tissue, Mel nodded. "I guess so," she said. "I just don't understand, Jenny... how could this happen? As smart as you are, and as much as you have going for you... what were you thinking?"

"Well, we made a mistake, Mom."

"You certainly did. And who's the other half of 'we' that made this mistake with you?"

Reaching into her purse again, Jenny pulled out her wallet, thumbed through it, and found a picture. "My boyfriend, Jeremy," she said, as she placed the picture in front of her mother. "I've mentioned him a few times to you, remember?"

Mel nodded. "I remember hearing his name once or twice over the phone," she said. "I just didn't realize that things were that... serious between the two of you." She studied the picture of her daughter's boyfriend, trying to grasp that the handsome, starry-eyed young man staring back at her would be the father of her first grandchild.

"We've been together for about six months," Jenny offered. "He's a junior, and he's majoring in business. He loves sports and his family runs a sporting goods store," she said.

Mel dabbed the corners of her eyes with a fresh tissue. "Have you told him yet?"

Jenny nodded. "Yes, of course. He was the first one that I told."

"And how does he feel about you being pregnant?"

"He told me he'll support me, whatever I choose."

Mel felt her stomach twist into knots. "It's not a choice, Jenny, it's a baby. Does he realize you're Catholic and that we don't believe-"

"Yes, Mom, we talked about all of this. We felt like our choices were to either keep the baby, or give it up for adoption."

"Do you really think you could do that, Jenny? Carry a baby for nine months and then adopt it out to another family?"

"No," she shook her head slowly. "That's why I'm keeping the baby."

"You're keeping the baby," Mel said. "What happened to 'we?' I thought you said he was going to be supportive of you, no matter what you chose."

"He did," Jenny assured her. "He says he'll be there for me and for the baby, and he'll support the baby financially, of course…once he graduates and gets a job and is able to do so."

"Is he going to marry you?" Mel blurted out.

Biting her lip, Jenny sunk back into her seat, distancing herself from her mother. "We're not sure that's the right thing for us right now, Mom. I mean, we've only been together for six months and he's still got one more year of college—"

"This isn't about you and him anymore," her mother interrupted loudly. "You're going to have a baby, for God's sake, don't you understand what that means? You have to do what's right for that child. You can't put yourselves and your own lives first. Neither of you can. Never again. You're bringing another person into the world, and that baby will always have to come first. Don't you get it, Jenny? Your life as you know it is over. It's OVER."

"No it's not," Jenny began to cry as she defended herself. "You were the same age that I am when you had me. Did you feel that way, Mom? Did you feel like your life was over because you had me?"

"It was different for me!" Mel almost shouted. "I was finished with school. And I was married to your father…."

"Dad's being totally supportive about this. So why can't you?"

Stunned, Mel sat up straight in her chair. "You told your father before you told me?"

"Yes," her daughter replied. "I told him last night."

"Why not me first?" Mel asked, her voice tightening.

"Because I knew you'd freak out," Jenny wept.

"I'm not freaking out," Mel said angrily.

"Yes you are."

"I'm not."

"I'm not going to argue with you, Mom," Jenny said.

Mel shook her head. They sat silently for several moments.

"When is the baby due?" Mel finally asked.

"In about five months. I'm taking the rest of the semester off. And the next one as well."

Mel felt as if someone shot ice through her veins. Her heart fluttered. "Five months? Jenny, how can that be? That would mean that you're about halfway through your pregnancy. You're not even showing yet. You don't have a belly..." but just as the words left her mouth, Mel took note of the bulky shirt that her daughter was wearing, and it suddenly registered that Jenny had simply been hiding behind clothing until she chose the right moment to break the news.

Mel began to tear up again. "Five months," she repeated. "Why did you wait so long to tell me?"

"I was scared." Jenny looked away ashamedly. "I knew you'd be disappointed in me. And I was right. You are."

No longer able to maintain her composure, Mel began to cry uncontrollably. She rested her elbows on the table and cupped her hands against her face, hiding her emotional display from the growing number of onlookers at the tables surrounding them.

"I can't," Mel finally said, when she regained her composure. "I can't deal with this right now, Jennifer." She stood and walked away from the table, abandoning her lunch, her shopping bags, and her daughter.

"Where are you going?" Jenny called out behind her, but Mel didn't answer her. Armed with only her handbag draped over her shoulder, she went for a walk around the mall.

What in the heck just happened? Mel wondered. *This isn't how my day off was supposed to turn out. Jenny and I were supposed to be walking around right now, looking for a gown for me to wear to the Dogwood Ball at the hospital next weekend. Jenny told me that she was coming home from college for an extended weekend visit. Not to tell me that she was pregnant and dropping out. That certainly wasn't part of the plan. Was it?*

As she brushed through the crowd of strangers on their shopping sprees, she watched their faces, feeling jealous of those who were laughing and smiling, or chatting happily with family or friends who walked by their sides.

Why do all of you people have to be so flipping happy today? She wondered. *My life just changed in the blink of an eye and nothing will ever be the same. I'm just barely forty years old and I'm going to be a grandmother. A GRANDMOTHER!*

Mel's stomach rumbled angrily at her for having walked out on her lunch. She spied a drink machine close by and stopped to pick up a soda. Searching in her handbag, she only found eight pennies and a quarter. Thankfully, the drink machine accepted credit and debit cards, so Mel dug into her wallet for her Visa.

It's a sad day in America when a person has to finance a canned soft drink on a credit card, she mused.

She swiped the card.

UNABLE TO COMPLETE TRANSACTION were the words that appeared on the LCD display above the card reader.

Mel looked down at the card and ran her thumb over the magnetic stripe on the back, hoping that it would fix the problem. She swiped again.

UNABLE TO COMPLETE TRANSACTION, still.

She checked the expiration date to make sure that the card was still valid. It was. Although her name wasn't.

Imelda Page, it said.

She hadn't been Imelda Page for more than a year. After the divorce, she switched back to her maiden name, Tagaro. To remove every trace of her ex-husband, Bruce, from her life, everything associated with him had to go. All of the property that they had shared – homes, cars and furniture and every little knickknack that they'd ever mutually owned – was gone. Their wedding anniversary was no longer a special day, and since it was only two days before Mel's birthday, she gave up her birthday too.

All she kept were their two children, Jenny and Michael. Ironically enough, as hard as she had worked to remove Bruce from her life, her two children were her daily reminders that he had been her partner for more than twenty years. Fourteen year-old Michael was a miniature version of Bruce. He had his father's wavy brown hair, strong jaw and dazzling smile. With the exception of Mel's slightly darker skin tone and just a hint of her almond-shaped eyes, Michael looked almost identical to Bruce in pictures of him at the same age.

Jenny was the exact opposite, drawing all of her physical appearance from Mel's side of the family. She and Mel were often confused for sisters, with their long, raven-black hair, that they both wore just slightly past their shoulders, the same eye shape and color, and same skin tone. Mel swore she could see in Jenny's pretty face hints of her own mother and sister, who she'd left behind in the Philippines when she'd moved to North Carolina twenty years ago. Yet Jenny's personality was a carbon copy of her father's. She was funny, charming and sweet at her best. And at her worst, she was maddeningly stubborn and a bit too impulsive at times.

Like four months ago, Mel thought, as she shook her head, still not quite ready to accept the fact that Jenny was pregnant.

Her stomach growled, and she tried to swipe the card one more time.

UNABLE TO COMPLETE TRANSACTION.

Great, thought Mel. *Now it's a sad day in Dogwood, North Carolina, when my very own credit card gets declined from buying a Diet Coke.*

Then she remembered. Just the week before, she'd finally swapped out the balding tires on her rusty Toyota Camry for new ones, with a hefty price tag of more than four hundred dollars attached. Since she'd just made a tuition payment for Jenny, her checking account was drained, so she'd pulled out the trusty Visa to cover the tire purchase. The statement had arrived in the mail a few days ago, but Mel had stopped looking at her credit card balances. She was too afraid of what she'd see. Apparently the charge for the tires had run the card up over its limit, and Mel suddenly felt horribly embarrassed for not having enough money to her name at the moment to buy a one-dollar soda.

She hadn't always had to struggle financially. Bruce had taken over the law practice after his father retired, right around the time that he and Mel got married. Bruce's career as an attorney in one of Dogwood's most respected law firms paid well, and they had lived comfortably. They certainly didn't need the extra income from Mel's job as a nurse, but she enjoyed the work. Even after Jenny and Michael came into the picture, Mel had found that she could still balance her duty to her family and her passion for nursing by simply cutting back to a part-time schedule.

When Bruce met Amanda over the Internet a few years ago and left his family for her, Mel was relieved that she'd never given up her nursing career and was thankful that she had the means to make it on her own. She refused alimony, even when it was offered to her, and settled on the first child support offer that Bruce made. Mel had been able to make ends meet for a long while, until Jenny graduated and went to college. Now that Jenny was past the age of eighteen, Mel's monthly child support checks were cut in half. And since Jenny had enrolled in college, the tuition bills were putting more of a financial strain on Mel than she had anticipated.

Bruce had offered to pay for all of Jenny's school expenses, but Mel's pride wouldn't let her accept. *Split them in half with me*, she had bartered back. No way was she ever going to give him the bragging rights to being the one parent who put Jenny through college. Once Amanda moved in, his attention – and his finances – suddenly had higher priorities than Jenny's education, so Bruce accepted Mel's deal without any protest.

Mel looked at the vending machine's hateful words once more - UNABLE TO COMPLETE TRANSACTION – and began to cry all over again.

If I can't buy a soda, how in the world am I going to be able to afford to help Jenny have her baby?

For a split second, she thought about calling Brad, her best friend from work.

But for what? She asked herself. She certainly wasn't expecting him to drop what he was doing and come to her rescue at the soda machine. She knew she could count on him for a shoulder to cry on over Jenny's news, but that could wait. Brad had confided in Mel earlier in the week that he was planning to pop the question to his girlfriend, very soon, if he hadn't already. She knew that this week would be a special time for both of them, and didn't want to rain on their parade.

Her stomach twisted into knots at the thought of a wedding.

It's Jenny who should be the next one in my life to get married. That stupid boy, Jeremy whoever, should have asked her to marry him the minute she told him the news. How committed can he be to his child if he's not committed to Jenny?

Then she thought about calling Bruce.

Looks like we're both going to be grandparents in a short while, so let's go ahead and get some things straight. At some point, I guess, I'll throw a baby shower for Jenny, and Amanda will NOT be invited. Oh, and there will be a baptism, too, and the both of you can sit that one out as well. I wonder how that's going to go over in church... an unwed mother bringing her baby in for a baptism and pledging to give the child a Christian upbringing? That should raise an eyebrow or two. I hold you personally responsible for this, Bruce. You're the one who set the example, by taking our marriage and your family so lightly. What were you thinking? When you put a ring on my finger and said "I do" and gave me two children to raise... did you think it was all just a big joke? Was it really that easy for you to walk away?

Mel suddenly wanted to scream out loud.

Stupid men! I hate you all!!!

"Looks like you're having a tough day," a man said softly from behind her. She whirled around to find her friend, David Carl, the Director of Pastoral Care at Dogwood Regional Hospital. "I came by the mall to pick up a birthday gift for my grandson, but I thought I recognized you and had to come say hello."

"Oh, David," Mel wept. "It's nice to see you." She reached up and blotted her eyes, suddenly feeling ashamed for her harsh feelings toward the whole male gender. David was possibly the most kindhearted person she'd ever met in her life, and had provided her with a great deal of support during the difficult months following her separation and eventual divorce. Mel had been hesitant to share too much with anyone else at work, for fear of confidences being broken and having her personal life broadcast to the rest of the world. It was already hurtful and embarrassing enough that her husband had left her for another woman, and the last thing that she needed was for her problems and her pain to become the latest material for the rumor mill at work.

David had been there for her on some pretty difficult days, and his office in the Pastoral Care Department had been her safe haven to vent, and to cry, and to help her hold onto her faith when everything else in her life seemed to be falling apart.

Mel forced a smile. "Sorry for being an emotional mess. This has just been such a horrible day."

"Well that's not good, considering it's only noon and the day is just getting started." He glanced over Mel's shoulder to see the cold words of electronic rejection blinking on the vending machine. "What can I do to make it better for you?"

She shook her head. "Nothing. I'm fine, really. Just having a hard day."

"Can I buy you a drink?"

She laughed. "I haven't had anyone use that line on me in years."

David chuckled as he pulled a dollar out of his wallet and fed it into the machine. "Lady's choice," he said, stepping aside for Mel to push the button for her selection. A Diet Coke dropped with a heavy thunk. Mel popped the top and sipped it. "Thank you so much," she said.

"My pleasure. Are you planning on going to the Dogwood Ball next weekend?"

She nodded. "Yes, I'll be there. Since I finally got a day off from work, my daughter and I came to the mall today to see if we could find any new dresses on sale, but no luck."

As in, no luck on having the funds to buy a new dress, Mel thought.

David glanced over her shoulder. "And where is your daughter?"

"Oh… she's at the food court, having a bite to eat right now. In fact, I should get back to her."

He smiled. "All right. I hope the two of you enjoy the rest of your day together."

Fat chance, Mel pouted. "Thank you, David."

"Are you sure you're going to be okay?"

"Yes. I'm fine. I just have a lot going on right now. Things I need to think through."

"Well, if you decide that it would help to have someone to talk to, you know where you can find me."

"Thanks, David. Say a little prayer for me, will you?"

"No," he shook his head, confusing Mel for a split second. "Only a BIG prayer for you, Mel."

She laughed. "Okay."

"I learned a long time ago not to be bashful about asking God for big things," he said. "If God can part waters, move mountains… you know, big things like that… then fixing our problems and healing our hurts can be a snap."

"I don't know," Mel shrugged. "It might just take a miracle in my case."

"Then that's what I'll ask for. And you do the same."

Nodding, she smiled and finished her drink. "Thanks, David. For the soda, and for just being there."

"Always Mel. Blessings," he said, as he waved and returned to his shopping.

As soon as he left, she felt a twinge of guilt.

Poor Jenny. I left her sitting alone in the food court. What was I thinking?

Mel rushed back to the table that she'd stormed away from only moments ago, to find Jenny with her face buried in her hands, crying.

"Jenny," she said softly, "I'm sorry, honey. Let's go. We can talk more at home."

Chapter 2
Tuesday
Donna

"Mom… I'm coming home."

Donna LeShay froze in her steps, nearly dropping her phone onto the kitchen floor. The voice on the other end of the line continued.

"I had my parole hearing last week, and I just heard back from the board today. I did it, mama. I made parole."

She took a deep breath and closed her eyes. As she was searching for the right words to say, she tried to exhale, but found that her throat and chest had tightened, making it nearly impossible.

Instead, she made a noise like the squeak of a tiny mouse.

"Mama?"

"Oh Darius!" she cried out, in almost a scream. The air from her lungs struck the mouthpiece of the phone with such force that for a long moment, only a loud static could be heard by either of them on the line.

"Mama, are you okay?"

Donna swallowed hard, blotted the tears that were springing from her eyes, and sighed. "I'm more than okay, baby. I'm wonderful. God has answered my prayers. You're coming home, at long last."

"I was hoping you'd be happy."

"Darius, I'm thrilled."

"You sound surprised."

"I am. I'm mostly surprised just to hear from you," Donna explained. "It's been almost a year. No phone calls, no letters, where have you been?

"You know where I've been, Mom."

"Well of course, I know where you've been. What I meant is where have you been as far as we were concerned – your family? You shut us out, baby. We missed you so much. We would have come to visit you if you had wanted us to. We wrote you so many letters I think we took down an entire forest with all the trees that were used for the paper. If there was any way we could have called you, we would have. We waited for so long to hear from you, Darius. What happened?"

He laughed softly. "I knew you wouldn't let me off the hook that easily, mama."

"You know not," she affirmed.

"I was busy getting my life together," Darius explained. "I was taking classes, going to some meetings here and there, getting involved in some good stuff for a change."

"Well son, that's wonderful! But were you really so busy that you couldn't find the time to call or write for a whole year?"

He hesitated for a moment. "I wanted to talk to you and Jeanette and Sean. I really did. I missed you all so much. But I was afraid that if I told you about what I was doing... going back to school and focusing my life on positive things... you'd get your hopes up, and if I somehow messed it all up, it would break your heart."

He paused, and his breathing suddenly seemed amplified, as if he were cupping his hand around the mouthpiece for privacy. "I've disappointed you so much that I didn't want to hurt you anymore. I didn't want to break your heart, Mama," he said. His voice tightened, and it suddenly became obvious that he was fighting not to cry.

"I love you, son," Donna choked out. "With all my heart. And the worst pain in the world was not having you in my life. Promise me you won't do that to me – to us – ever again. Good news, bad news, school or screwing up, prison or parole, it doesn't matter. I need to hear your voice and see your face, or else I'm not a whole person. Do you understand?"

He sniffled loudly. "Yes, Mama," he replied. "I'm sorry."

"It's okay," she said. "You can make it up to me as soon as you're home. In fact, I'm looking at a tower of dirty dishes in the sink right now that have your name written all over them."

"Well, I've washed plenty of dishes here in prison," Darius laughed. "I never thought I'd actually get excited about being able to wash dishes at home."

"So when do you get out? Do I need to come pick you up?"

"I need you to come to the prison tomorrow, if you can. You'll have to fill out some papers before I get out. I have to have a sponsor – someone who can guarantee me a place to live without any drugs or alcohol in the home, and you'll have to be willing to let my parole officer come to the house to check up on me from time to time."

"I think I can handle that," Donna said. "As long as YOU promise not to bring any drugs and alcohol into my home. I'll have some terms and conditions of my own, son, and you know me, I'm going to be tougher than any parole officer could ever be."

"You have nothing to worry about," Darius assured her. "I'm a different man now, Mama. We have a lot of catching up to do."

"It sounds like it."

"So tomorrow then?"

"Sure. Where do I need to go once I get there?"

"There's a two story brick building that's right there by the highway, you can't miss it. It's the only one not enclosed in the twenty-foot high fence. That's where you'll go. Just walk in and tell them you're there to pick me up and they'll get you to the right place."

"Okay, I think I can handle that."

"Oh, Mom?" Darius paused for a moment. "You're coming alone, aren't you?"

"Yes. Your sister will be in school tomorrow and your brother is living in Chapel Hill now, at the University."

"Oh, good," Darius sighed. "I just… wouldn't want them to see me here."

"Well they know where you are, Darius," she said. "It's not like it's a big secret."

"I know," he said. "But I don't want them to see me behind bars. Not even for a minute, not even walking out of here."

"Why?"

"Because that's where the old Darius belongs – behind bars. I'm leaving the old 'me' here for good. I'm walking out of this place a new man, who's going to be a better son, a better brother, and a better person in every way. You'll see, Mama."

Donna took a deep breath again, and exhaled. "I can't wait to see you, son."

"Tomorrow at ten?"

"I think so. I'm supposed to work tomorrow, so let me call in and see if I can make some arrangements for coverage. It's not as easy to get time off once you're the boss," she said with a laugh.

"The boss? For real?"

"For real. I'm a nurse manager now, on the Med-Surg South Unit. Have been for almost two years."

"Wow," Darius murmured. "Congratulations, Mama. We've got a lot of catching up to do."

"Yes, we do. And it's a long drive back from Raleigh to Dogwood, so we can start when I pick you up. Unless I send word that I can't get away from work tomorrow, I'll see you then."

"Drive safe, Mama."

"I will, Darius."

"I love you."

"I love you too."

Chapter 3
Wednesday
Haylie

"Mom, I'm moving out!" Haylie Evans was beaming with pride. "I found a new apartment. It's in that little complex, Dogwood Park, the one that they just built last year, near the hospital. It's so close, I can literally walk to work now, Mom. Isn't that cool?"

Joann, Haylie's mother, stared back at her daughter. "Are you sure you're ready for this, honey?"

"Ready or not, here I come!" Haylie giggled as she bounced up and down on the sofa and clapped her hands. "I just signed the lease, on the way home from work today. I put down the security deposit, and they gave me the keys."

"Oh," Joann said, trying not to sound too disappointed. "That's great, honey. I just thought we were going to go apartment hunting together."

Haylie looked chagrined. "Well... yeah, that was the original plan, but I made a new friend at work today. Her name is Jaime and she's a new nurse on Med-Surg North. She's about the same age as me. We were a bit short-staffed on the unit today, so they sent Jaime to the South side to help out. Well, she and I really clicked, and then we went to lunch together. She was telling me how she just leased a new apartment with her boyfriend in Dogwood Park, and how much they love living there !"

"Oh Haylie," her mother interrupted her, "Dan's not moving in with you, is he?"

She grinned. "No, Mom. Relax. Just because Jaime lives with her boyfriend doesn't mean I'm moving in with mine. I haven't even told Dan yet. We're not making any plans to move in together."

"Good," Joann sighed with relief. "You know I like Dan a lot, honey. It's nothing against him. I just… you know, don't want to see you rush into something like that."

"I promise you, Dan and I are absolutely not moving in together. I wasn't even thinking about him when I leased the apartment."

"So… how exactly did you arrive at that decision?"

"Well, I told Jaime that I was looking for an apartment. I told her how I've been living at home since I started working at Dogwood, about a year ago, and saving up my paychecks so that I could build a little nest egg before getting a place of my own. And I told her how you and I have been talking about starting to look for an apartment, and how I've got a nice amount of money saved to go ahead and make the move."

"Right," Joann nodded.

"So, Jaime was telling me about Dogwood Park and how great it is. There's an Olympic size swimming pool, and a tennis court, and water and trash disposal are included in the rent. Plus, every tenant gets two parking spots, and you know the best part of all? There's a lighted footpath straight to the hospital, and a security call station midway, so it sounds totally safe. And it's only a five minute walk, or even quicker by bike. Isn't that cool?"

"Extremely cool," her mother agreed.

"Anyway, Jaime said that I could come look at her apartment if I wanted to get a better view of the complex. So I did. I walked home with her and took at look at her place. It was so awesome, Mom! She has walk-in closets! And a huge bathroom with a Jacuzzi tub!"

"It sounds nice," her mother agreed.

"Oh it is. So right after I talked to her, I went to the leasing office. They showed me three open units, and I picked my favorite one, which just happens to be in Jaime's building. They ran a credit check on me and had me sign a lease agreement, and I wrote them a check for the deposit and first month's rent. And then…" Haylie paused for effect, as she reached into her handbag and withdrew a set of keys. "They gave me the keys to my new place. So it's official. I've got my own home!"

"Congratulations, sweetheart." Joann picked up the keys and ran her fingers over the grooves, trying to fathom that this was really happening. Her youngest daughter was moving out, and she would finally have an empty nest. She wondered what it would be like to live alone for the first time.

Then she wondered what it would be like for Haylie to live alone. "Are you thinking about getting a roommate to help share the rent?"

"Heck no. This is going to be my place and my place only. Do you think I'd give that up so quickly?"

"I guess not," Joann shrugged.

Haylie's voice took on a dreamy tone. "I'll finally get to watch whatever I want on TV, and can stay up as late as I want with all the lights on, and I can play the radio as loud as I want, and I won't have to worry about anybody else! This is going to be my own little place, my very own home, and I can't wait!"

"Well congratulations then," her mother smiled. "Will you at least let me come over and help you decorate? Help you pick out some furniture and curtains, maybe?"

"Of course," Haylie said, springing to her feet and circling her mother in her arms. "I'd love for you to help me out. And hey... what about you? Now that I'm moving out of my room, are you going to do something fancy with it? I love what you did with Isabel's room when you turned it into another family room. I think we spend more time in there now than we do the living room."

Joann gave a half-hearted smile. "Not sure yet, Haylie. I think I'll probably just leave it the way it is for now. Just in case..."

Haylie looked offended. "In case of what? Trust me, Mom, I won't be moving back home."

"Just in case things don't work out. You never know, Haylie. What if it turns out that the apartment complex isn't as safe as you think it is, or living on your own gets too expensive? I just want you to have another option."

"That's sweet, but I'm going to make it work, one way or the other."

"Well, your room will still be here, just in case."

"Mom!" Haylie said in a huff. "When Isabel got married last year, you didn't give her the 'just in case' speech, did you?"

"No, of course not."

"So don't 'just in case' me either."

Joann suddenly looked as if she might cry. "I'm not trying to hurt your feelings. I just want you to know that you'll always have a home here, honey. You're my baby, you know, and I sometimes can't believe that you've grown up."

"Oh Mom, you're such a mush." She squeezed Joann's hands.

"I'm proud of you, Haylie. You're a beautiful young woman, and you're smart and kind and hard-working, and you're the best nurse that Dogwood Hospital has on staff, even if you've only been there for a year."

"I am so not the best nurse at Dogwood," Haylie protested. "But thanks for the vote of confidence."

"You know I'm your biggest fan, don't you? And always will be."

Haylie grinned. "So bring my one-woman fan club into my bedroom and let's start packing. What do you say?"

Chapter 4
Thursday
Brad

"Susan Elizabeth Chase, will you marry me?"

Brad Jackson dropped to one knee as he spoke the words, and pulled a velvet-covered clamshell jewelry case from the breast pocket of his suit jacket.

He'd been saving up for nearly a year for the ½ -carat diamond solitaire ring. He would have waited a bit longer and gone for a full carat, but in prior conversations with Sue, she had insisted that she didn't want a big stone. "You don't need to spend your life savings to impress me," she had assured him. "I'd be happy with a plastic ring from a gumball machine. It's not about the price tag or the size of the diamond... it's what the ring represents."

He expected to see her sparkling green eyes beginning to tear up, and he was absolutely certain that she'd be grinning from ear to ear with her signature gorgeous smile.

Instead, she was biting her lip and staring blankly ahead.

She's in shock. Give her a minute, Brad told himself. He waited a little while for the transformation to occur. His knee was getting sore.

"Brad," she began, "I... I really don't know what to say."

He stood up and sat down at his seat, staring at her from across their table in La Fiesta, their favorite Mexican restaurant.

"I picked the wrong place, didn't I?" Brad sighed.

Some might have thought it tacky to propose during happy hour in a Mexican restaurant, but Brad thought it was only fitting. After all, it was where he and Sue had dinner on their first date. Six months later, it was where they went to celebrate Brad finishing nursing school and getting a job at Dogwood Regional Medical Center. A few months after that, it was where they decided that they were ready to move in together, and pored over apartment listings for hours to find their new home. A year later, it was the place where they'd suffered a nasty fight in which Sue dumped a pitcher of margaritas over Brad's head and broke up with him because she was convinced he would never ask her to marry him. The breakup didn't last long, though, and after a couple of weeks of being apart, they met there again for dinner and decided to work things out, with marriage as a possibility someday.

Surrounded by the smell of fajitas, the bright lights and colorful ponchos hanging on the wall, and the sounds of a mariachi band playing for tips in a distant corner of the restaurant, Brad suddenly began to wonder if he should have picked a more romantic venue to ask his girlfriend such a life-altering question.

"No, you didn't pick the wrong place," Sue assured him with only a shadow of a smile. "It's just that I really wasn't expecting this. You caught me off guard."

He breathed a sigh of relief. "So now that the surprise is over, can I get a 'yes' and a kiss from my fiancée?" He looked at her hopefully.

Sue fanned out the fingers on her left hand and flexed them, watching the diamond capture and scatter light with each movement. "Oh Brad," she whispered. "I wish I could say yes. But I can't." She hesitated for a moment before slipping the ring off of her finger. She placed it in the palm of his open hand.

He stared at her, waiting for an explanation.

"I know that I pressured you and pushed you to do this," she began, "and I was wrong. I'm so sorry. I know you're probably pretty upset with me, but I hope you'll be able to forgive me someday."

"But… but I thought this is what you wanted," Brad murmured as he slid the ring back into the clamshell case. He wanted to feel something. Angry, sad, he wasn't sure. All that he could muster was confusion.

"I thought it was too," Sue said. "And had you asked me a year ago… probably even six months ago… maybe even three months ago, I would have said yes. But it would have been a mistake."

"A mistake?" He looked up at her, filled with a new kind of hurt that he'd never before experienced in his life. "Why?"

Sue reached across the table and took his hands into hers. "I know this is going to be hard for you to understand, Brad, but it's time for me to move on."

He sat back with a jolt. "Wait a minute… you're breaking up with me?"

"I had no idea you were going to ask me to marry you," she defended herself. "I swear, Brad, I had no clue. I was going to tell you tonight about my plans."

"What plans?"

Sue took a deep breath. "You remember me telling you about my sister?"

"You mean Sandra? The one who's doing mission work at the orphanage in Croatia?"

She nodded. "Yes. I'm going to join her."

Brad stared blankly at her. "You're moving to Croatia," he said.

"Yes."

"Just like that. You're just going to pick up and move?"

"Well… not exactly. I had to apply to the same outreach program that she's in, and I had to wait until I heard back from them that I was accepted. And I've been taking some online classes in child development. And I had to get my passport, of course…"

"And how long did all of this take you?"

"A few months."

"And why am I just now hearing about this?"

Sue hung her head. "I wanted to wait until I knew for sure that I was going to get accepted, and that it was all going to work out."

Tracing the outline of the jewelry case with his fingers, he sighed loudly. "So I guess this means it's a done deal, right? You're going?"

She nodded. "I leave in two days."

"For how long?"

"A year, at least," she said. "Maybe longer. I don't know yet."

He sat silently for a moment. "I wish I had known sooner," he finally said. At last, the anger and the sadness were starting to set in.

"I'm sorry," Sue offered. "I guess part of me was afraid you'd try to talk me out of it. Or that you'd propose to me in hopes of keeping me here."

"And why would that have been such a bad thing? Don't you love me?"

She smiled. "Brad, of course I love you. This isn't about you. It's about me."

Brad sighed deeply. *I've used that line lots of times*, he thought. *Never dreamed it would come back to haunt me.*

Sue leaned forward in her chair and rested her elbows on the table. "For the past four years, I've been working as a sales clerk in a gift shop, Brad. I don't have a job like yours. You get to help people every single day. I want to know what that feels like."

"So stay here. Go to nursing school, and you can come to work with me at Dogwood when you graduate. We could always use another nurse on Med-Surg South."

She shook her head. "That's not what I want, Brad. I've chosen my own path."

"But why Croatia? Why do you have to go so far? Aren't there some underprivileged kids here in North Carolina you can help?"

Sue reached into her purse and pulled out a photo of her sister Sandra, kneeling down in front of the remains of a burned-down building, surrounded by children in very plain-looking clothes. She slid the photo across the table to Brad.

"I remember seeing this," he said. "Your sister mailed this to you like... months ago."

"I know," Sue said. "And I've been looking at this picture every day since she sent it to me. That building in the background was the orphanage that the kids lived in before it was destroyed in the war. The kids have been living in the basement of a church since then. Sandra's part of the team that is rebuilding a bigger and better orphanage for them. And in the meantime, they're teaching the kids English, and they're helping American and British parents adopt those kids. They're really changing those children's lives, Brad."

He watched her face light up as she spoke. Her eyes were sparkling with passion, the kind that he had hoped to see only moments ago when he had proposed to her.

"I want to be a part of that," Sue continued. "Every time I talk to Sandra, she always tells me about the great things that they're doing, but how they could do so much more if they had more people to help. So I'm going to do that."

He nodded slowly. "Okay," he said. "Okay. If that's what you want to do, then you should do it."

Sue smiled. "I was hoping you'd understand. I feel as if a weight has been lifted off my shoulders." She sighed deeply.

"So you'll go and spend a year there, maybe a little more, and then you'll just come back to Dogwood, and we can just pick up where we left off, right?" Brad looked down at the jewelry case again.

Sue's smile quickly faded. "I don't know," she said.

"Well then I'm confused," Brad quickly responded. "Because just a minute ago, you said you loved me. If you love me, and I love you, then a year apart won't change that, will it?"

The shimmer of passion left her eyes as quickly as it had appeared, and was replaced by the deepest sadness that Brad had ever seen. "Brad, I don't know. I don't know what's going to happen in a year's time. Maybe I'll want to stay in Croatia. Maybe I'll come back home and we can start all over again. I have no way of knowing what's going to happen. That's why I don't feel like it's fair for me to make any promises to you right now."

They sat in silence until their server came to take their dinner order.

"I think I'm going to pass on dinner," Brad said.

"Me too," Sue said.

Brad dropped a few dollars on the table and walked out of the restaurant. Sue followed at his heels.

"Brad... wait! I know you're hurt, but don't you want to talk about this?"

"No, I don't. Let's just go home. I'll help you pack."

They didn't exchange a single word during the journey home. Once inside their apartment, Brad opened the closet door in the hallway to the living room to hang up his jacket. He spied the tuxedo that he'd purchased a few weekends ago.

Brad thought back to the first time that Sue had seen it.

"What's that for?" She had questioned him, when she'd first seen him wrestling the long suit bag from the men's formal wear store into the closet.

"Well, you're going to love this," he'd said, as he rolled his eyes playfully. "I got recruited for the bachelor auction at the Dogwood ball. It's part of their fundraising campaign for building the children's hospital. The unit or department with the bachelor that brings in the highest bid wins a weekend at the beach in a luxury condominium. Mel and everyone else on first shift asked me to volunteer for it since I'm the only guy on the unit who's still single… I mean, still technically single because I'm not married." Then he paused, and with a smile, added "Yet."

It was the first time that he'd shared the news of the bachelor auction with Sue, and he was hoping for a reaction of some sort. Perhaps a small joke about being jealous, or a spirited comment about her attending the ball with him and saving up her money to bid on a date with him. Or maybe even a comment about the tux, followed by a question about when he intended to wear it again. And for what occasion.

Instead, she had merely smiled and told him what a kind gesture it was.

Thinking back to that day, it finally dawned on Brad why she hadn't taken the bait. He shook his head as he sank down onto the sofa, wondering how he could have been so clueless.

Sue sat down on the loveseat opposite from him, and for a long while, only silence filled the space between them. She sniffled and wept. Brad wanted to do the same, but fought the overwhelming urge to cry. Still, Sue's tears were wearing down his resistance, and he finally joined her on the loveseat. He wrapped his arm around her in an effort to comfort her, and ultimately prevent his own breakdown from occurring.

"I don't want you to be mad at me," she said.

"I'm not," he said. "All I ever wanted was for you to be happy. I asked you to marry me because I thought that's what you wanted."

"It was, a while ago," Sue confessed. "And maybe someday, it will be again. But not right now. I'm sorry."

"You don't have to be sorry. I love you and I want you to be happy. So... if this is what you want, then it's okay with me. Go without any regrets."

"You promise... you're not mad?"

"No," Brad said truthfully. "I'll admit I'm confused... and sad, but no, I'm not mad."

"I'm sad too," Sue sniffled. "You have no idea how hard it's going to be for me to say goodbye to you."

So don't, he wanted to say, but instead pulled her close and gave her a kiss on the cheek. "You'll be alright," he assured her. "You're stronger than you realize."

Apparently much stronger than I am, he said to himself. The unfamiliar ache in his chest grew more intense. Without even thinking, he cupped his hand over his heart, searching for the steady beat beneath his fingertips to let him know that it was still there, still beating, and hopefully not as broken as it felt at this moment.

Chapter 5
Friday
Miriam

"It's a boy!" Miriam Simpson shouted with excitement as she stepped off of the elevator and onto the Med-Surg South nursing unit. "Seven pounds and four ounces, with rusty red hair and the chubbiest little cheeks you've ever seen!" A photo was in her hand.

Miriam was the senior nurse among all others on Med-Surg South. She held more than thirty years of nursing experience, having spent twenty-two of them at Dogwood Memorial Hospital, in a wide variety of settings and units. However, when she'd been assigned to Med-Surg South eight years ago, she finally felt like she'd found her home as a nurse, and it was just where she wanted to stay until the day she retired, which she'd planned to do the prior year. But then her husband, who had been ill for quite some time, passed away.

Miriam and her husband had one son, Brandon, who had moved to California years ago for a job with a prestigious engineering firm. When he bought a house in his new hometown and married Jessica, a fellow employee at his firm and a California native, Miriam knew that she wouldn't be seeing much of him anymore. Her prediction had been correct, as she'd seen Brandon and his wife only four times during the past twelve years. Three of those times had been during holidays, and the last had been for his father's funeral.

After the funeral, she found that her house was eerily quiet, and the weight of loneliness was far too much to bear at the time. Miriam would wake up each morning excited about going to work, and dreading the thought of coming home at the end of the day. Her colleagues had taken the place of her family now.

Donna, the nurse manager, was the warm and wise mother figure of the unit, even though Miriam was more than ten years her senior. Haylie was Med-Surg South's newest nurse, and Miriam had been assigned as her preceptor when she arrived. Although the differences between them had been vast and they got off to a rocky start, they had smoothed things over, and Miriam soon began to think of Haylie as the daughter she'd never had. Mel and Brad were the other two nurses on the unit whose work ethic and skills Miriam deeply respected, and whose company she truly enjoyed. She thought of them as her sister and brother.

In spite of her allegiance to her new family, Miriam began to question delaying retirement when Brandon moved back to Dogwood ten months after the loss of his father, with Jessica, who was eight months pregnant at the time.

She had gone into labor just the night before, and Brandon had called Miriam en route to the hospital. She joined them in the delivery room, where she tearfully witnessed the arrival of her very first grandchild.

"It's a boy, it's a boy, it's a boy!" Miriam announced again, breathless with excitement.

Haylie, Brad and Donna immediately abandoned whatever they were working on at the nurse's station and gathered around Miriam to see the picture of the new arrival.

"Isn't he gorgeous!" Donna said, prying the picture out of Miriam's hands for a closer look.

"Cute little fellow," Brad agreed.

"He sure is. What's his name?" Haylie asked.

"Timothy Brandon," the proud grandmother responded, carefully enunciating each syllable of the baby's name as if the words were somehow sacred. "They were going to name him after his late grandfather, but I asked them not to. For obvious reasons." She cocked an eyebrow and smiled.

Years ago, Miriam had worked as a Labor and Delivery nurse, and had often wondered what parents were thinking when they chose names for their children. Some of the names that she had seen appear on birth certificates were purely comical, like the one that had been chosen by basketball-loving parents, Mr. and Mrs. Duncan. They had named their baby boy Slam Duncan.

Some names were just plain outrageous. The baby girl born to a Miss Charlotte Sedan had been named Luxury. Luxury Sedan.

Unlike those parents who had purposely given their children those unusual, attention-getting and sometimes just plain ridiculous names, her late husband's parents had named their son with none of the same intentions.

His mother came from a newly immigrated family of Greeks. When she met the very American Mr. Simpson, it was love at first sight, and they were married shortly thereafter. When the new Mrs. Simpson found out that she was expecting, she pondered the implications of raising her son in her new American house, with an American father and all of his American customs governing the home. Hoping to imprint some of her Greek heritage forever into her son's life, she insisted on giving him a legendary Greek name. It was just very unfortunate for him that she settled on Homer, the Greek poet, as her child's namesake. And so he was named – Homer Simpson.

Of course, there was no way to foresee that a cartoon character of the same name would be created several years later, and that it would have found such a stronghold in American pop culture.

"I would never have forgiven them, had they named him after his grandfather," Miriam laughed.

"You should tell Mel that they did name him after Homer," Brad said. "See how long it takes her to figure out you're just joking."

"That would be funny, but mean," Miriam grinned. "I'm too excited to be mean right now. Where is Mel, anyway?"

"Here I am," Mel announced, appearing from a patient's room and joining the small crowd gathered around Miriam.

Mel took one look at the picture, and her smile faded. "Congratulations, Miriam," she said. The color drained from her face as she spoke. "He's a beautiful boy. Really."

Miriam wrinkled her brow. "You look like you just got hit by a truck. What's wrong with you?" She asked Mel. "I mean, I know I'm prejudiced since I'm the kid's grandmother, but sheesh, he's not that bad looking, is he?"

"No, Miriam. He's a beautiful little boy."

Miriam studied the picture more closely. "Are you sure? I mean, I know his face is sort of wrinkled up in the picture, but I think that's just because he was constipated—"

"Oh stop. He's adorable. I promise." Mel forced a smile.

Miriam studied the picture. She looked worried. "You'd tell me if I had an ugly grandkid, wouldn't you?" She began to sound worried.

Mel finally laughed. "Miriam, I swear to you, your grandson is absolutely perfect."

"So what's up with you then? The look on your face when you saw his picture was horrid. If you could have seen it yourself, you'd know what I was talking about."

Shaking her head, Mel shuffled away. "It's nothing, really. I'm just not feeling great today."

Miriam, Donna, Brad and Haylie exchanged curious glances. "Something's up with her," Miriam said with conviction. "Go talk to her, Brad. She'll let you know what's going on."

"Don't push her," Brad objected. If she wants to talk about it, she will eventually. If she doesn't, you'll never hear a word. That's just Mel."

"That's not healthy," Donna said, shaking her head with worry. "It's not good to keep things all bottled up inside."

"Well, maybe she'll find someone else to confide in," Brad said. "Maybe she just doesn't want to broadcast her personal life at work."

Miriam nodded. "That's always a possibility."

"Well, if you don't mind me changing the subject, I have some news," Haylie said proudly. "I just leased a new apartment yesterday, and I'm moving in over the weekend. I've got my own place to live now! The rent is reasonable, it's a brand new unit, and it's a five minute walk from work. How awesome is that?"

"Congratulations!" They said to her, almost in perfect unison.

"And I have good news to share too," Donna smiled. "Darius got out of prison and came home on Wednesday. That's why I took the last two days off, to be with him."

"Congratulations!" Miriam, Haylie and Brad said, almost in perfect unison once again.

"So much to celebrate," Miriam said excitedly. "Donna's son came home, Haylie just got her first home, I have my first grandchild… and Brad, what about you? Any big news from you?" Miriam looked at him expectantly.

He simply shook his head. "Sorry. No news here."

"So you haven't popped the question to Sue yet?" Haylie asked.

He looked away. "Yes, I popped the question." An awkward pause followed. "I just didn't get the response I was looking for. She's decided to do something different with her life. She's moving to Croatia to work on a mission project with her sister in an orphanage."

"Oh…. I'm sorry," Miriam apologized.

"It's okay." Brad said with a shrug. "I'll live." He forced a smile and left the group, making his way toward a patient room.

"Open mouth, insert foot," Miriam scolded herself. "I never saw that coming. I thought for sure Sue would have said yes. Now I feel horrible for bringing it up."

"It will be okay," Donna assured her. "There don't seem to be any hard feelings from Brad's end, so don't waste any time beating yourself up. Not when you have that handsome new grandson to be so happy about."

A smile spread across Miriam's face as she looked at the baby's picture again. "He is pretty handsome, isn't he? His grandpa sure would be proud."

Chapter 6
Saturday Night

"Tickets please, have your tickets ready, please!" Bellowed out a sweet-faced elderly lady, whose voice made her seem much larger than her petite frame. She reached out her hand, causing a ripple in the royal blue sequins of her gown that started at her sleeve and shimmered to the hemline grazing the floor.

"Here you go, Ms. Benson." Brad handed her five tickets, one for each person at his table. "I almost didn't recognize you. I'm used to seeing you in your pink volunteer coat, scooting around the hospital behind a wheelchair. I gotta say, I think blue suits you much better than pink."

She blushed, kissed the tips of her fingers, and tapped them on Brad's cheek. "Thank you, darling," she replied sweetly. "I don't get many excuses these days to dress up, so I was just thrilled to snag one of the volunteer jobs at the Dogwood Ball. And you're looking mighty sharp tonight, if I say so myself."

Brad looked down at his tuxedo and smoothed the lapels of his jacket proudly. "Why, thank you, Ms. Benson. You do know I'm up for auction tonight, don't you?"

"Of course! I've got my checkbook AND my credit cards, and don't think I wouldn't max them all out for a date with my favorite nurse. Unfortunately, I don't think I stand a chance, my dear. My daughter is coming to the ball tonight, too, and she spotted your picture in the marketing posters for the Dogwood Ball. She already told me that you're her top choice."

Brad grinned. "Well if she's as lovely as you, I don't think I'd mind her winning a dream date with me at all."

Ms. Benson cocked an eyebrow. "You'd have a lot more fun with me!" She insisted.

"Well then good luck with the bidding." Brad laughed as he took Ms. Benson into his arms for a bear hug.

"Awwwwwwww!" His four colleagues cooed in unison behind him.

"Too cute, Bradley," Mel said, nudging him from behind. "But would you mind letting us squeeze past you? We're all starving for dinner!"

Miriam, Haylie, and Donna nodded in unison.

"Go ahead, young man," Ms. Benson said, patting him on the back. Go enjoy the evening with your entourage of lovely ladies!"

"Thanks Ms. Benson!" Brad grinned and stood to the side to let his co-workers pass in front of him. "Ladies first."

When the nurses entered the conference room, they were stunned to see the transformation. Each of them had been in the room a number of times for events like employee orientation, committee meetings, uniform sales, required trainings and the annual safety fair, but never before had they seen it like this.

The sterile room with white walls and endless tables and chairs had been magically transformed for the Dogwood Ball. Round tables were scattered about the room, covered in white and pink tablecloths. The lighting was low, but candle centerpieces ringed with white dogwood bouquets provided enough lighting for everyone in the room to appreciate the beauty and splendor of the evening. Helium filled balloons and streamers covered the walls and the ceiling. A deejay was spinning records on a parquet dance floor in the middle of all of the tables, and at the far end of the room was a raised platform with a podium and a catwalk for the bachelor auction. And all around them, their fellow hospital employees were meandering around, nibbling on hors d'oeuvres and admiring each others' formal wear.

"It's like high school prom," Haylie said, her eyes sparkling with memories.

"It's like the military ball, my last year in the Navy," Brad said softly, reminiscing his days in uniform.

Donna blinked rapidly. "This reminds me of the big surprise party that they threw for my Sean at church in the fellowship hall, when we found out that he got accepted at UNC."

Mel sighed. "This room looks a lot like the place where we had my... my..." she hesitated a moment, then finished her sentence. "My wedding reception." She forced a smile, but the sadness was apparent in her eyes.

Donna placed a sympathetic hand on her shoulder. "We're going to have a great time tonight," she reassured her with a smile. "And we'll make lots of good memories. The kind that you'll want to hold onto forever."

"Yeah," Mel agreed. "I know we will."

Moving as a unit, the five nurses wove through the rows of round banquet tables until they found the one with a card perched in the middle of the floral centerpiece, bearing the words "Welcome Med-Surg South."

"Guess this is us," Donna said, waving her staff toward the table. She waited for all of them to take their seat, and then planted herself at the chair in the middle of them, much like a mother on an outing with four young children.

Shortly after they were seated, a jazz quartet took the stage and began to play a breezy, lighthearted song to set the stage for the evening. Servers in tuxedos suddenly appeared around the perimeter of the room with massive trays on their shoulders, and began serving salads and dinner rolls. Then the hospital CEO, Richard Jorgenson, took the microphone.

"Welcome, everyone," he began with gusto, "to Dogwood Regional Medical Center's annual Dogwood Ball!" The hundreds of Dogwood employees in the room and their guests applauded in response.

The CEO continued. "Thank you all for joining us for this very special event. The evening will be filled with music, dinner and dancing, and the best part, our bachelor auction!" Thunderous applause filled the room, punctuated with cheers and shouts, whistles, and high-pitched "wooohoos!" from the ladies in the audience. Several of the women in the crowd pushed back their chairs and stood up to show their enthusiasm.

Laughing, Mr. Jorgenson waited for the crowd noise to die down. "Can all of the bachelors please take the stage at this time?"

In response to his request, twelve of Dogwood's single male staff, all dressed in tuxedos, rose from their seats throughout the room and made their way toward the stage. They included three male nurses, two respiratory therapists, three residents, one physician, a pharmacy technician, an accountant from the hospital's finance department, and even a local celebrity of sorts, a retired Senator who served on the hospital's board of directors.

The bachelors lined up on stage, triggering more applause and excited shouts from the female portion of the audience. Donna, Miriam, Haylie and Mel cheered Brad on as he took his place in the lineup.

Mr. Jorgenson continued. "We'll begin the bidding shortly after dinner. The highest bidder for each bachelor will win a dream date of the winning lady's choice. One hundred percent of the proceeds from the auction will go toward the building fund for the new children's hospital." More applause filled the room. "As many of you know, the closest children's hospital is nearly one hundred miles away from Dogwood. We desperately need one of our own in this community, so that we can care for critically ill children close to home, and alleviate the burden of costly and time-consuming travel for their families. Our children deserve this, and Dogwood Regional Medical Center is going to make it happen!" Everyone applauded, including the bachelors onstage.

"It's going to take millions to make the children's hospital a reality, and we're starting tonight. Our goal is to raise ten thousand dollars in our Bachelors Auction. So bid high and be generous, ladies," Mr. Jorgenson encouraged the audience, then turned to the bachelors. "And gentleman, we're counting on you to charm every lady in this room into opening her heart... and her checkbook... for this good cause." Laughter erupted throughout the room. Each of the bachelors smiled and struck a pose.

"Brad looks pretty good, doesn't he?" Mel asked Haylie, nudging her with her elbow.

"Yeah he does. The tux does him justice," Haylie replied.

"If only I were a rich woman, I'd bid on him," Mel said with a little laugh.

"Yeah, but what would be the point? He's your best friend. You guys hang out all the time anyway. If you wanted a dream date with him, all you'd have to do is ask."

Mel rolled her eyes. "I was going to say, I'd bid on him and give the dream date to you as a present. He's like my kid brother, Haylie. I couldn't go out on a date with him!"

"And neither could I, I've got a boyfriend now, remember?" Haylie looked over her shoulder at the cluster of tables set aside for the Emergency Department staff and locked eyes with Dan, an Emergency nurse, and her boyfriend of nearly a year. He smiled and winked at her.

"Yeah, yeah," Mel grinned. "I like Dan. But Brad is cuter. I think you and him would be great together."

"Oh Mel... don't start this again. Just because Brad and Sue broke up doesn't mean you're obliged to play matchmaker."

"I'm just kidding, Haylie, relax," Mel laughed.

Miriam jumped up from her seat and slid into Brad's vacant chair next to Mel, inserting herself into the conversation "Well, all joking aside, I'm hoping one of us from Med-Surg South will bid on him and win, because there's someone else who's got her eye on him that I think may do it if we don't."

"Who?" Mel asked, jumping into the conversation.

"Cassandra Putnam," Miriam whispered.

"Cassandra Putnam?" Mel blurted loudly.

"Shhhh!!!" Miriam and Haylie scolded her in unison.

Donna cast them a dirty glance, "Quiet!" She mouthed to them.

"Cassandra Putnam is Dr. Putnam's wife," Miriam said, ignoring her boss. "And she's got quite a reputation around here." Miriam arched an eyebrow.

"What do mean?" Mel asked.

"Man-eater," Miriam nodded. "Nothing but trouble, that one. I've seen her come around the hospital under the pretense of visiting her husband, but she conveniently shows up when he's in the middle of a surgery, or isn't around. So she hangs out and flirts with the other docs instead. She likes them cute and young. Loves the residents. And male nurses, too."

"I hope I don't hear what I'm hearing," Donna whispered. "That sure sounds like gossip to me!"

"Gossip? Me? Never," Miriam said sweetly. Mel and Haylie simultaneously kicked her under the table.

"So where is Mrs. Putnam?" Mel asked, craning her neck to glance around the room.

Miriam jerked her head a couple of times to the right.   "Two tables down. Do you see Ms. Benson? She's sitting right next to her."

"Oh my," Mel shuddered.

Cassandra Putnam was obviously in a solid state of denial that she had passed the age of forty. As well as thirty. Twenty, even. She was squeezed into a purple halter gown that Mel recognized from her trip to the mall the weekend before. Specifically, it was the dress on the mannequin in the window display at the juniors-only dress store in the mall. Her long bleach-blonde hair swung behind her in a ponytail, and was adorned with sequined butterfly clips.   From behind, she could have easily been confused for twenty-two year old Haylie. It wasn't until Cassandra turned slightly to the side that Mel saw her face and got the full effect.

"Wow," was all that she could say. "Her lipstick looks like clown makeup."

"Those fake eyelashes look like tarantulas." Haylie said, completely mesmerized.

"They sure do." Miriam murmured softly. "Wonder who did her makeup... the funeral home?"

"Miriam!" Donna snapped from across the table. "Stop being so mean!"

"You're right," Miriam said, pretending a look of shame. "It was pretty mean for me to suggest something like that about the funeral home. They made Homer look so much better than Mrs. Putnam before I buried him."

Haylie and Mel doubled over in laughter, drawing unfriendly glares from surrounding tables.

"I mean it," Donna said with authority. "Cut it out."

"Alright, alright," Miriam relented. "But just to let you know, I did see her checking out Brad earlier in the lineup. She walked past him and winked, and then made an obscene gesture."

"What kind of obscene gesture?"

Miriam began to raise her hands above the table.

"No, wait… don't show me. I don't want to know." Donna put her own hand up in a "stop" gesture and looked away.

Miriam shrugged. "Suit yourself. But just wait till the bidding starts," she said. "She's going to go after poor Brad with a fury. Bet you anything."

"So what? Let her bid and win him. The money's all going to a good cause."

"Sure it is," Miriam agreed. "But is it really worth it to sacrifice our poor Brad in the name of making a buck for the hospital?"

"Sacrifice is a strong word," Donna growled. "It's just a date."

"Uh huh," Miriam said in a low voice. "Take a look at her and tell me if you think she just wants a date."

They glanced at Cassandra Putnam once again. She was pointing at Brad, winking suggestively, and licking her lips.

Mel's eyes grew wide. "She's right. We have to save him!" She dug into her handbag and pulled out her wallet, flipping to her checkbook. She thumbed through the pages of the register until she found her balance. "I've got… fourteen dollars," she said with a sigh.

Haylie shrugged. "Don't look at me. I'm broke. I just paid a huge security deposit on my new apartment and put down payments on a new living room and dining room set at the furniture store. I'm tapped out."

Donna looked at Mel sadly. "Sorry," she said. "I just took Darius out last night and spent a ton of money on clothes for him. We went a little overboard, since it's the first clothes he's been able to wear in years that don't have "Department of Corrections" stenciled on them."

Miriam arched an eyebrow. "This could get interesting," she said, playfully.

Groaning, Mel stuffed her checkbook back into her purse and tossed it under the table. "Poor Brad," was all that she could muster.

Dinner was served shortly thereafter, and Mel pushed her vegetarian lasagna around on the plate with her fork while her co-workers feasted on filet mignon and chicken cordon bleu. She was dreading the bachelor auction, and was wishing that she hadn't encouraged Brad to volunteer for it. She felt like a failure, knowing that she had no means to rescue him from the very predatory-looking Cassandra Putnam.

When Richard Jorgenson took the podium once again to start the Bachelor Auction, Mel's stomach flip-flopped. The respiratory therapist was the first one up for bid.   He strutted down the catwalk, flashing a dazzling smile and winking at the woo-hooing ladies as he passed. He brought in a bid of eight hundred dollars. An excited young woman that Mel didn't recognize was the lucky winner.

Next came one of the residents. Tall, dark and hairy, with a long ponytail and thick beard and mustache. He reminded Mel of a caveman. However, there was something about the way that he smiled and sauntered down the catwalk that told Mel that his personality made up for what he lacked in looks.   The bidders became a bit more aggressive, and the lucky winner was a nurse anesthetist that won him for a little more than two thousand dollars.

The next couple of residents were only moderately handsome. One of them brought in five hundred fifty dollars; the other brought in just under nine hundred.

Next came the retired Senator, who brought in a winning bid of nearly three thousand from the Director of Rehab Services.

And then it was Brad's turn.   He smiled as he strutted down the catwalk, completely unaware of the fate that awaited him.   Mel looked over at Cassandra Putnam, who already had her checkbook in her hands, and looked as if she might start foaming at the mouth at any minute.

Mr. Jorgenson read a short description of Brad to entice the bidders. "Our next Bachelor is Brad Jackson, who was born and raised in St. Louis, Missouri, and found his way to North Carolina by way of the Navy. Brad completed a four-year tour of duty as a medic, and finished his service at Camp Lejeune. Brad then moved to Dogwood, and worked as a paramedic for Dogwood EMS for two years. Then he decided he was ready for a career change, and went to nursing school. He came to work for us at Dogwood Regional Medical Center when he finished school, and has been one of the stars of the Med-Surg South Unit ever since. Brad is bilingual and speaks Spanish fluently, which puts him in high demand on his unit whenever there's a Spanish-speaking patient. In his spare time, Brad enjoys playing golf, working out and playing video games. Let's start the bidding for Brad at two hundred dollars."

Cassandra Putnam shot out of her seat. "How about two THOUSAND?" She cried out, obviously uninterested in the fanfare of a bidding war. Lots of applause followed her comment, and she glanced around the room to see if there would be any contenders. Much applause followed.

Brad squinted to see past the bright stage lights shining in his face, following the sound of her voice. When his eyes focused on Cassandra standing up and waving her checkbook like a flag, he gritted his teeth together and waved back.

"Oh my God," Mel whispered to Miriam, breaking out into a sweat, "I think he just saw her. Did you see the look on his face? Poor Brad…"

"Don't give up hope just yet," Miriam said.

"Wonderful! Mr. Jorgenson said, smiling. "It looks as if we may just exceed our ten thousand dollar goal tonight! Two thousand dollars is the current bid for Brad Jackson. Do I hear two thousand, five hundred, perhaps?"

And then, as if on cue, another woman rose from her seat in the far corner of the room. "Here!" she offered.

The room was filled with "ooohs" and "aaahs."

"I know who that is. She's a nurse practitioner from one of the local family practices," Miriam said, as she craned her neck to get a look at the challenging bidder. "Looks about Brad's age. Very cute. A saucy little redhead – he'd like her, I bet."

Mel breathed a sigh of relief.

"Two thousand, five hundred," Mr. Jorgenson said, pointing at the nurse practitioner.

"THREE thousand!" Cassandra shouted, without missing a beat.

More ooooh's and aaaaah's from the crowd.

"Three thousand," confirmed Mr. Jorgenson. "This is our highest bid yet. Would anyone care to top three thousand?" He paused for a moment. "Going once, going twice…"

"Three thousand… two hundred," the nurse practitioner piped in, still playing along, but obviously nearing her threshold.

"Three thousand, five hundred," Cassandra immediately shot back.

"Three thousand... seven fifty," the nurse practitioner said, a little more timidly.

"Four thousand," Cassandra grinned.

"Four thousand!" Mr. Jorgenson cried out with delight. "Going once, going twice... do I hear any bids above four thousand? Last chance..."

"Five thousand dollars," bellowed out Miriam, rising from her seat. "Five thousand dollars, over here!"

Everyone in the room gasped as all eyes turned toward her. Mel nearly fell out of her chair. Surprised gasps, laughter, and applause filled the room.

Cassandra opened her mouth to top the bid, but before any words came out, Miriam shouted, "Oh heck, let's just double that and make it ten. Ten THOUSAND dollars!"

Cassandra did a double take in Miriam's direction. "E... eleven... thousand dollars!" She shouted toward Mr. Jorgenson. It was obvious that Miriam's bid had caught her by surprise.

"Twelve thousand," Miriam shot back.

More applause.

"Thirteen," Cassandra squeaked out.

"Thirteen thousand," Mr. Jorgenson said with gusto. "Going once, going twice—"

"Oh, what the heck," Miriam cried out, "Let's just make it an even fifteen thousand."

Cassandra's face turned ghostly white, and she sank back down into her chair, obviously defeated. Ms. Benson patted her shoulder and whispered a few words of consolation into her ear.

"Fifteen thousand dollars," Mr. Jorgenson said loudly and slowly, drawing out each syllable. "Going once! Going twice! SOLD!"

Every person in the room simultaneously rose to their feet, applauding and cheering in Miriam's direction – including Brad, who was wiping the sweat from his brow as he stepped down from the stage.

"Miriam, I can't thank you enough!" Mel said, throwing her arms around her. "Are you sure you can afford fifteen thousand dollars?"

Smiling, Miriam nodded. "Homer left me a small fortune. My salary is just play money at this point, so I've been socking my paychecks away in a savings account. I figured I may as well pull some of that money out and support a good cause. Or two, in this case. Helping fund the building of the Children's Hospital, and rescuing Brad from Cassandra Putnam."

Brad rejoined them at their table. He hugged Miriam as soon as she was freed from Mel's embrace, and thanked her with a kiss on the cheek. "I can't thank you enough," he said with a sigh of relief.

"No problem, Brad. But did you happen to see that cute little redhead that put in a couple of bids for you?"

"Just barely. I had bright lights in my face the entire time I was on stage."

"Well you should go and talk to her. She's adorable. And obviously quite interested in you. In fact, I was thinking of doing yet another good deed and donating my dream date with you to her. I bet you'd have more fun on a date with someone your own age than me."

Brad shook his head. "No way," he said with a grin. "You won the date fair and square, Miriam. So you name the time and the place, and we're going out on a date." He put his arm around her again and pulled her to his side. "I'm all yours, so you better get your fifteen thousand dollars' worth."

Miriam raised an eyebrow. "Okay," she said. "Tomorrow then."

"What time?"

"All day long. I'll pick you up at eight o'clock in the morning."

Brad looked at her curiously. "Alright," he said, laughing. "An all day dream date with Miriam. I couldn't imagine a better way to spend a Sunday."

"Dress for comfort," she instructed him. "Nothing too glamorous. Ditch the tuxedo for sure."

***

Mel struggled to keep her eyes open as she drove home. Once

inside of her apartment complex, she parked, retrieved her mail from the mailbox, and pulled off her high-heeled shoes for the upstairs climb to her home on the second story of the complex.

As she ascended the flight of stairs to her apartment, Mel sifted through the mail and strained her eyes, trying to salvage the last bit of faint daylight in order to read the fine print on the envelopes in her hands. Pizza coupon, postcard from uniform supply store, utilities bill, car insurance bill, Jenny's tuition bill for the upcoming semester...

She stopped as she reached the top of the stairs and sighed deeply. "Stupid bills," she muttered under her breath.

"Who's Bill?" A deep, male voice blurted out suddenly.

Startled, Mel looked up from her stack of mail and gasped in surprise. Upon seeing the unexpected visitor waiting at her doorstep, she instinctively stepped back to distance herself from potential danger. Losing her footing on the stairwell, she shrieked and began to fall.

"Whoa there!" The visitor lunged forward and grasped her by her arms, pulling her forward. "Are you okay? I'm sorry, I didn't mean to scare you."

Mel steadied herself and brushed his hands off of her. Moving quickly past him, she retrieved her keys from her purse and headed for her door. "What do you want, Bruce?"

He was quiet for a moment. "Well hello to you, too," he said, not attempting to hide the sarcasm in his voice. "And you're welcome."

"Welcome? That's interesting. I didn't know that I had anything to thank you for in the first place." She whirled around, shooting him a stern look.

"I kept you from falling down the stairs, didn't I?"

"I wouldn't have fallen had you not been standing here in the shadows like some kind of stalker. What do you want?"

He stepped closer toward her. "I just came to talk, Mel. We haven't talked in a while." He reached out and took her hand into his. "There are times when I just... I don't know, Mel... I guess I kind of miss the way we used to talk. And I miss you. I miss us. I just wanted to talk to you again, to see how you're doing."

She snapped her hand out of his grasp, as if his words had

delivered an electric shock. "Are you kidding?" Mel could feel her cheeks flush with anger. "Go talk to your trophy trade-up fiancée. I'm done talking to you."

Mel opened the door to her apartment, stepped inside, and slammed the door.

Bruce knocked immediately.

"Go away!" She commanded from the other side.

"Imelda, please. Are you going to hold a grudge forever? I just want to talk to you."

"GO AWAY!" She yelled.

"Five minutes. That's all I'm asking."

Silence.

And then, the knob twisted and the door opened. Mel faced her ex-husband with her arms crossed and her eyes lowered to her watch. "Five minutes. Right here in my doorway. And then you go. If you're not gone after five minutes, I'm calling the cops and they can escort you away."

Bruce looked hurt. "Cops? Are you serious? I'd never lay a finger on you. Why would you call the police?"

"I asked you to leave, and you didn't. You're now officially trespassing on private property, and that's a crime." She looked down at her watch. "Four minutes and fifty seconds."

"Alright, alright," he said. "Mel, I don't want it to be like this. I don't want us to NOT speak to each other. Can't we just forgive each other and move past everything?"

She looked up at him, her eyes flashed with anger. "Forgive each other?" Her voice rose slightly. "Pray tell, what do you have to forgive ME for, Bruce?"

"Well, that's not what I meant. I guess that didn't come out right."

"No, Bruce, it didn't. Enlighten me as to what I did wrong? Did I drive you to cheat on me with that tramp in your law firm? Or did I push you to log onto the Internet to find the lust of your life, Amanda? Did I fail you at marriage counseling somehow? I showed up for all of the sessions. You quit coming. Hah! My goodness, what was I thinking? How inconsiderate! Can you ever forgive me, darling?" Mel's voice had risen to almost a shout. Her arms unfolded, and she clenched her hands into fists at her sides.

Bruce retreated a step. "Calm down, Mel. I know you're mad at me, but if you don't take this down a notch, it will be your neighbors calling the cops."

"You still haven't told me what you want, Bruce. Don't tell me you're here to talk."

"Mel," He began, then hesitated. He took several deep, loud breaths through this mouth as he collected his thoughts. He seemed distressed.

She looked at her watch again. "Less than four minutes now. You're wasting my time if you're just going to stand there panting like a dog. But oh, how appropriate is that? You ARE a dog."

"Okay. You want to know why I'm here? Because I get it now. I finally get it. I made a mistake, Imelda. I screwed up, and I realize it now. And I'm sorry."

She wasn't expecting this. Never in a million years would she have expected this.

He continued. "I know that what I did to you - to our family - was wrong, and I'm sorry, Mel. I am so sorry."

She blinked several times. She partly expected tears, but she wasn't too surprised when they didn't spring freely from her eyes.

Bruce boldly stepped forward again, grabbing Mel by the shoulders. "I want to try and work things out with you. For us. For the family."

Mel looked him in the eye, searching. For what, she wasn't sure, but she suspected that she'd know it if she saw it. Truth? Hope? The promise of a second chance?

But all she could see was the man who had betrayed her.

"You've got great timing, Bruce. You do realize that you had lots of chances to 'work things out,' long before you walked out on me, don't you?"

He nodded. "Yes. I know I had a lot of chances to get it right, and I blew every single one of them. All I'm asking for is one more. Just one last chance, and I promise you, Imelda, never again. Never again will I hurt you. I promise I'd be there for you, and I'd be good to you. For the rest of our lives."

Unconvinced, she shook her head again. "You made some promises to me before God and all of our friends and family on our wedding day. You didn't keep any of those. Why start now?"

"What do I have to do?" He begged. "Please... please. Can you at least just think about it? I'd go back to counseling, and I'd show up for every single appointment, I swear to you. I could get it right this time."

Mel rolled her eyes and leaned against the door frame. "How does Amanda feel about all of this?"

Upon the mention of his fiancee's name, Bruce clammed up. The passionate expression on his face faded and was replaced by a look that reminded Mel of the way that her patients grimaced in post-op pain. He had no answer for her.

"What about Amanda?" She asked again. "How does she feel about all of this?"

"Mel... it's not that easy."

"So you haven't shared this with her," Mel interrupted. "You haven't dumped her, have you?"

"Don't call it dumping. That sounds so childish."

"Hah!" Mel laughed loudly. "Childish? That's what I call it when a grown man goes slinking back and forth from one woman to another, trying to make certain he's got a sure thing lined up before he ditches one for the other."

"I'll tell her. I promise you. It's just that now is not a good time—"

"Get out of here, Bruce," Mel demanded. "You're a scumbag. Get out of here and never come back." She disappeared behind the door and slammed it in his face.

"Imelda!" He yelled. "Come on... don't do this! We're going to be grandparents!"

Mel flung the door open again, with enough force to rip it off of its hinges. "Don't you dare throw that in my face," she hissed. "Jenny and her baby have nothing to do with us."

Advancing forward, Bruce put his foot in the doorway. "We're not getting any younger. We're going to have a grandchild. Amanda's not old enough to be a grandmother. She's barely old enough to be a mother. And she wants to have kids with me! I can't do that! I can't have a son or a daughter younger than my own grandchild!"

Mel narrowed her eyes. "All things you should have thought about before you threw your family away on a twenty-something fantasy girl."

"Mel, please."

Her stare pierced him like a dagger. "Tell you what, Bruce," she began, "since you've grown a conscience and you want to do the right thing, I'm going to give you a chance."

He advanced forward a step. "Anything, Mel. Anything."

"You and I are through. There's no point in trying to change that. But your daughter needs you. Now that she's not going to be a full-time college student anymore, neither of us can carry her on our health insurance. So she's going to have a very costly labor and delivery bill at the hospital. And then she's going to need baby clothes and food and diapers and the whole nine yards. She'll probably need childcare at some point, whenever she decides to go back to school, or else goes to work. I'm not expecting much out of the father of her child, and I can't afford to do it all on my own, Bruce. I'm working myself to death and I'm still barely able to make ends meet for myself and our two kids. So if you want to help me, and Jenny, and your grandchild, you can open up a savings account and start adding money to it every chance you get."

The color quickly faded from Bruce's face, and his eyes widened.

"What," Mel said in almost a growl. It was a demand, not a question.

"I'm having some financial problems myself."

Mel bit her lip. *This isn't happening,* she said to herself.

"Mel, I can't," he simply said. "Amanda's not the person I thought she was. She has a bit of a … spending habit. She's maxed out all of my credit cards, and things are so bad at home—"

"And if you're expecting sympathy from me, I'm terribly sorry, but I've got none to give. Now get out of my apartment, and out of my life."

"Imelda! I love you! Doesn't that mean anything?"

"I told you to get out. Doesn't that mean anything? Apparently you're having a hard time finding your way, so let me help you." She kicked him in the shin and he jumped, stumbling backward down the stairwell and dropping onto his rear end at the concrete landing. "Owww!" He cried out.

"You're welcome!" She screamed, and slammed the door.

Inside, Mel found Jenny sitting cross-legged on the floor in front of the television. She made her way to the living room and crashed on the sofa.

"Dare I ask what happened between you and Dad?" Jenny looked over her shoulder at Mel.

"Your idiot father," Mel replied in a huff. "He really has some nerve to show up here after everything he's done."

"I figured you'd feel that way. That's why I wouldn't let him in when he knocked on the door earlier. I thought you'd probably kill me if I did, so I told him to wait outside." Jenny sighed deeply. "You know, Mom, I really wish you and Dad could just move past all of your issues. It's hard being caught in the middle of it sometimes."

Mel ignored the latter part of Jenny's comment. "Well, you did the right thing. Except for the part about telling him to wait at the doorstep. You should have told him to fling himself off of the stairwell and land on his head on the concrete below."

Jenny shook her head and rolled her eyes. "Whatever, Mom. So what did he want?"

"He wanted to talk," Mel said, as she rolled up her eyes.

"About what?"

"Should you be sitting so close to the TV?" Mel asked, shifting the conversation in a new direction.

"Why do you ask?" Jenny looked confused.

"The baby, Jenny…"

"Mom," Jenny scolded her, "The TV isn't going to hurt the baby. What do you think is going to happen, anyway?"

"You never know. I just think it's better to play it safe."

Jenny shrugged. "I don't know what's unsafe about the TV. Other than... I don't know..." Her tone suddenly became very serious. "Maybe... dangerous radio waves beaming in from the satellite in outer space that are going to penetrate my belly and turn the baby into an alien? And me too?" She curled her fingers until they looked like claws and raised them up on either side of her face. "Mom... you were right! It's happening! The aliens... they're taking over my body through the television.... Aghhhhhhhhhh!!!" She opened her mouth widely and began to drool on herself.

Mel rolled up a magazine on the coffee table and whacked Jenny on the shoulder with it. "Quit it," she commanded. "You're not funny."

"Everything's going to be fine."

"Well I don't know about that," Mel snapped. "All of that horrible stuff on TV these days... violence and sex and drugs and cussing... I would hate for the baby to hear all of that and think that's what it's going to be like out here in the world. I'd never want to be born."

Jenny turned up the volume to drown out her mother's voice.

"Good evening, I'm Tammy Smith," announced the perky blonde news anchor. "And I'm Jim Raynor, and this is the eleven o'clock news" chimed in her slightly balding, but still made-for-TV handsome co-anchor.

The camera zoomed in on Tammy and she flashed a dazzling grin. "Thanks for joining us," she cooed. "In tonight's news, Hollywood comes to the small town of Dogwood. Mayor Stephen Rice and several citizens of Dogwood officially welcomed the A-list cast and crew of an upcoming action movie to town today. They began arriving shortly after noon in vans, buses, campers and eighteen-wheelers hauling large pieces of equipment, in preparation for filming the movie."

Tammy's smiling face disappeared from the screen and was replaced by footage of the convoy she had just described. The camera captured each large vehicle, one after the other, as they passed by in a near blur.

"Highway 210 hasn't seen this much traffic in ages," commented an unseen male narrator. "And residents of Dogwood weren't about to miss out on all of the excitement. Spectators lined the highway today, cheering and waving as the movie crew made its way into town."

The camera zoomed in on the face of an elderly man wearing a baseball cap that said I love BINGO. "I ain't never left Dogwood in my whole life," the man said, with a thick Southern accent. "And I don't reckon I ever will. This may be my only chance to see someone from the picture shows live and in person."

Then a little boy with large, ill-fitting glasses and buck teeth appeared on the screen. He was sitting in a lawn chair on the shoulder of the highway, next to his mother and a couple of siblings. "Devin Ryan is like… my hero," he said nervously into the microphone. "I've watched all his movies. I can't believe he's filming the next one here in Dogwood!"

The unseen reporter across from him moved the microphone a bit closer to the boy's face. "So if you could meet him in person, what would you say to him?"

The little boy's face lit up. "Oh man! I'd probably just ask him for an autograph and I'd tell him he's the best actor ever. And I'd tell him that he's my hero!"

Jenny turned around and looked at her mother, wide-eyed with wonder. "Did you hear that? Devin Ryan is in town!"

"Heard it loud and clear," Mel said, unimpressed.

"Mom," Jenny nudged her mother's knee. "Don't you know how famous he is? He's starred in more than a dozen action movies. You and Dad took me and Michael to see some of them when we were kids. Remember?"

Mel's face soured at the mention of Bruce. "Yes, I remember."

"The last one we saw together… oh, I can't remember the name of the movie, but it was the one that was about the drug smugglers, and Devin Ryan was an undercover agent, and he saved that kidnapped girl and they fell in love. Do you remember, Mom? We went out for pizza that night. And all of the servers came and clapped and sang the birthday song, and we had to stand up and do the dorky clap-clap sing-a-long thing, remember? Whose birthday was it?"

"Mine," Mel said with a sigh. "It was my birthday."

"Speaking of, it's coming up again soon. What do you want to do to celebrate?"

Mel glared at her. "I don't celebrate my birthday anymore. You know that."

"Oh come on, Mom. That's stupid."

"No, it's not."

"Let's go out next weekend. Pick the nicest restaurant in town and we'll go and have dinner."

"With whose money?" Mel asked bitterly.

"I've got some. Not much, but enough to pay for a nice dinner."

"You should be saving every penny you can get your hands on right now. You're going to have some mighty big expenses coming up, you know…"

"Oh come on, Mom. Let's just go out! How about that nice new Italian restaurant – Bella Cucina – the one that just opened a few weeks ago downtown? I hear it's the hot new place to go for dinner on the weekends. Who knows, maybe we'll even run into Devin Ryan downtown and we could get his autograph!"

"Sounds fantastic," Mel said, with sarcasm dripping from her voice. "That would just fulfill all of my birthday wishes, to run into a no-talent moron actor like Devin Ryan."

Jenny spun around and faced her mother. "Could you please just lighten up for a change?"

"Now is not a good time to tell me to lighten up, Jenny. I've had a hard week. I just found out this week that I'm going to be a grandmother. I'm so broke I can't even buy a can of soda. I'm tired and I've got to work tomorrow since I'm picking up every extra shift I can to make ends meet. And now I'm worried about how we're going to pay for your baby to be born, and get by each month with another mouth to feed… do I need to go on?"

Jenny sat in silence for a long moment. Her eyes began to well with tears. "Well I'm sorry I ruined your life," she finally said. "And mine too, I guess."

Mel took a deep breath. "Jenny," she began, "Stop saying things like that. You haven't ruined anyone's life."

"Maybe I should just leave," she said. "I can move in with Dad and Amanda—"

"Stop," Mel said. "I'm not in the mood for a pity party. We'll get through this, but I'll be honest, Jenny, it's not going to be easy. This is going to change all of our lives."

"I know. Don't you think I'm freaked out and scared too?"

"I can imagine you are." Mel paused. "You're going to have to do a lot of growing up, really fast. And you'll be missing out on a lot of things, and giving up a lot of experiences that you would have been able to have, had you made different choices."

"Like what? What do you think I'm going to be missing out on, Mom?"

Mel glared at her. "I don't know, Jen, and I guess you never will either. All those things that you wanted for yourself... you can forget them now. Remember the summer trip to Europe that you were saving up for? Or the internship you were hoping to get in New York City during your senior year? Or just finishing college... how are you going to do that? You can't go to class toting a baby on your hip. And you can forget about going to football games and spring break trips..."

"Mom, stop!" Jenny cried. "I've already beat myself up enough for the both of us. I don't need to be reminded of what I'll be missing out on. I'm just trying to be positive now. And I really need your support."

"And I'm trying to give it to you, Jenny, I really am. I'm just having a hard time coming to grips with this. Give me some time."

"I know you're mad at me, Mom. And I know that I dropped a bomb on you. Maybe I didn't go about doing it the best way, and yeah, the food court at the mall was probably not a great place to have the talk. I guess I just felt ready at that moment and the words came out before I could really think about it."

"It's okay," Mel said. "Look, it's been a long day, and I'm exhausted, so let's just call it an evening. Once I get some rest, we can sit down and talk some more."

"Okay," Jenny agreed. "So if you don't mind a change of subject, how was the ball?"

"It was fun. Miriam put a fifteen thousand dollar bid on Brad and won a date with him."

Jenny's face finally brightened to a smile. "That's a riot," she laughed. "What about you? Did you win a bachelor?"

"Heck no. I didn't even bid."

"Mom! Why not? I saw the pictures of the bachelors in the newspaper yesterday. There were some total hotties in the mix!"

"No money. Do I need to remind you? Besides, I'm not interested in hotties right now," Mel grumbled as she rose from the couch and stepped into the kitchen. "I could go for a hot dog, though." She opened the refrigerator in search of a snack.

"Soy dog," Jenny corrected her. "Those things are gross and don't even come close to tasting like a real hot dog, so don't go insulting a perfectly good meat by-product by lumping it in the same category as your nasty soy stuff."

"Since when have you been eating meat?" She asked Jenny, shooting her a look that could kill.

"Since I went to college and finally got to buy my own groceries, after spending my childhood under the oppressive rule of a vegetarian mother," Jenny joked.

"Ughhhh, Jennifer," Mel sighed, slamming the refrigerator door shut and slinking into one of the kitchen chairs. "Really? You abandoned your veggie roots that quickly?"

Jenny got up from the sofa and joined her mother at the kitchen table. "Not really. I started eating meat after I found out I was pregnant. I had an appointment for bloodwork at the Student Health Center at school, and they told me I was anemic. They told me to try eating red meat. So, I did. And I have to tell you, Mom... I like it."

Mel sighed. "That's fine," she said. "You're entitled to call the shots for your own life now, I guess. I just wanted you and Michael to be healthy and eat only the best foods, and I thought that going vegetarian was the right thing for our family. Out of all the people that I ever took care of after coronary bypass surgery, I never once met a vegetarian among them."

"Yeah, and I appreciate you doing that for us, Mom. I have to admit, though, it was always tough to sit at the same table as Dad and watch him mow down pork chops while the rest of us nibbled on tofu and soy."

Mel glared at her. "Your father did love those pork chops. It's very true what people say... you are what you eat. And he's a pig, for sure."

"Mom!" Jenny snapped at her. "You're so mean."

"Why are you always so quick to defend him?" Mel retorted.

"Because he's my Dad," Jenny insisted. "You picked him, not me."

Mel crossed her arms. "I'm glad you love your father and I think it's very kind of you to be so loyal to him. But let me just say this, Jenny, I hope that when you fall in love and get married, it'll be forever. I hope no man betrays you and rejects you the way your father did to me. I hope you can at least understand why I feel the way I do. He hurt me, Jen, and it's going to take time to heal from it."

"I'm sorry about what Dad did, and I know it can't be easy for you, Mom," Jenny relented somewhat. "But it's been two years since he left. Don't you think it's time to move on?"

"And what makes you think I haven't?"

"I just want you to be able to let go of all that anger and be happy again."

"I am happy," Mel insisted.

"I mean the kind of happy that can't be stolen away at a moment's notice, by something like the mention of Dad's name or the sight of his face."

Mel looked at her smugly, not wanting to admit that Jenny had a point. "I'll get there someday."

"Sooner than later would be better," Jenny said, smiling slightly. "And I've been thinking… it would be kind of nice if you found someone else, you know?"

Arching an eyebrow, Mel leaned forward. "Have I been talking to myself all this time? Did you not hear a word I've said? Men are pigs."

"You said Dad was a pig."

"He is."

"Dad's not the only man in the world. All I'm saying is that it might be nice for you to get out there and start dating again. You don't need to spend the rest of your life alone, Mom. Surely there's going to be someone else who could make you happy."

"Not interested right now."

"You're afraid to move on," Jenny said, boldly. "Because if you did, then you might just get over being mad at Dad, and you might find out that it's not so horrible to forgive him and move on. The only one holding you back from being happy again is you."

Mel felt as if someone had dumped a bucket of ice water over her head. For a moment, she was too stunned to speak. "Jennifer, if you weren't pregnant, I'd open the door and toss you down the stairwell. Don't ever speak to me like that again." Mel stood up and made her way to her bedroom, slamming the door loudly behind her. Crashing onto the bed, she buried her face into a pillow and resisted the urge to scream.

She's wrong, Mel told herself over and over again. *Jenny's just a kid still, she has no clue. She's wrong, wrong, wrong about me.*

Still, she asked herself if there had been any truth to what Jenny had said.

Am I lying to myself?

She agonized over that question until the wee hours of the morning. Then she cried herself to sleep.

Chapter 7
Sunday

Brad baited the hook for his line, and then Miriam's. She cast hers into the water first, then he followed. With a couple of soft *plunks*, their lures sunk far below the surface of the water.

"Good job," said Miriam. "For someone who claims they don't know how to fish, you're getting the hang of it nicely."

"Thanks," Brad replied, grinning. "When I was in the Navy, we did some survival exercises. They put us out in the middle of nowhere and let us live off of the land for a few days. I caught a fish then and it fed a few of us dinner."

"How did you catch it? The Navy didn't drop off some fishing poles for you, did they?"

Brad reeled in his line a little. "Nah, they didn't. We had to figure out how to do it on our own. With nothing but our bare hands. That kind of thing."

"Oh, so you caught a fish with your bare hands? I'm impressed."

"Well…. I sure *tried* to catch a fish with my bare hands," Brad confessed, "but after doing that for a couple of hours with no luck, what I finally ended up doing was taking off my cammo's and trapping one in the leg of my pants."

"Are you serious?" Miriam grinned.

"Yeah," Brad said. "And it earned me the nickname 'Fishpants' for many years to follow."

Miriam doubled over with laughter, nearly capsizing the rowboat. "Well since you used to so lovingly call me 'Large Marge,' can I call you 'Fishpants' now?"

Brad scowled at her while he clinched his fishing pole between his knees and grabbed the sides of the boat, attempting to steady it. "Oh, you better not," he said.

"How about..." Miriam snickered, barely able to finish her sentence, "How about SpongeBrad Fishpants?" She howled with laughter again, and dropped her fishing pole. Brad caught it as it hit the water, just before it started to sink.

"Yeah, yeah," he said with a grin. "See if I ever tell you any of my cool Navy stories again."

Dabbing at her eyes with her sleeve, she finished up her laughing fit and took the pole back. "Well I didn't mean to mock you. Of course, you have to admit, it's kind of funny. Who would've thought that you could catch a fish with your pants? That's pretty unconventional."

"That's one way of putting it," he agreed. "I was hungry. Hadn't eaten in two days, so I did whatever it took to catch a fish."

"Of course," Miriam nodded. "That's what survival is all about."

"Exactly. When things are taken away from you, you learn how to adapt. You learn how to move on and keep living."

They sat in silence for a little while. On the horizon, the sun began to dip below the water's surface. It cast a warm, orange glow across everything, for as far as the eye could see. Brad pushed his sunglasses up off of his face and rested them on his forehead to appreciate the beauty of the moment.

"You know something, Miriam?"

"Hmmm?"

Brad turned slightly toward her. "It was really good to hear you laugh like that."

She chuckled again. "Yeah, I enjoyed it too. Are you sure I can't call you Fishpants?"

He touched her shoulder and whispered in her ear, "Only if you keep it just between us. Don't tell anyone at work, and for God's sake, don't tell the fishes."

"Oh, consider it our little secret, Bradley Fishpants," Miriam whispered.

After another brief moment of silence, Miriam sighed. "I miss this. I didn't realize how much I missed it until just now."

"Fishing, you mean?"

"Yes. As soon as the weather got warm, Homer and I used to go fishing every spring at this very lake. From the first year that we met to right up until the year he had his first stroke." She paused and pointed at the pier several feet ahead of them.

"That's where he proposed to me, Brad. Right there, at the very end. I think some of the wooden planks at the end have rotted away now, and a couple of the beams have collapsed into the lake, so the exact spot where he did it probably isn't there anymore, but that's still the same pier. That's where it happened."

He strained his eyes to make out the details of the pier. "Yeah," he murmured, trying to envision a lovely young Miriam, and handsome young Homer on bended knee before her.

She sighed loudly. "And I sure do miss that old codger."

Then Brad felt a pull on his line.

Miriam watched as the tip of Brad's pole was tugged downward toward the water. "You've got one," she said. "Start reeling it in. Not too fast, now."

Following her guidance, Brad reeled the line in. The pull from below the water's surface was growing stronger, and he could feel the fish fighting against him. His pole was tugged from side to side as the fish flailed below the water's surface.

"Steady," Miriam coached him. "A bit faster now. I'll get the net."

Brad reeled the line in until at last, a large silvery fish emerged, flailing wildly from side to side. He jerked the line back sharply toward him, and the fish landed with a heavy thud in the boat.

"What a beaut," Brad said proudly. "Even if we don't catch another one today, he's big enough for both of us to eat for dinner."

Miriam looked at him with contempt. "Are you kidding? That's the ugliest fish I've ever seen. Put that poor thing out of its misery. Take the hook out of his mouth and throw him back in."

Confused, Brad shook his head. "Are you serious? You want me to throw back a perfectly good fish because he's ugly?"

"Oh, they're all ugly out here, Bradley Fishpants." She picked up the fish and skillfully removed the hook from its mouth, then tossed it back into the water. The fish hit the water with a heavy *plunk*, and whipped its tail around on the surface for an extra few seconds, splashing Brad and Miriam as if to show his offense at being plucked from his habitat for no apparent reason.

"That was painful to watch," Brad lamented. "The first legitimate catch of my life, not involving my pants, and you just had to go and throw the fish back."

"It's called 'catch-and-release fishing,' Brad. Didn't you get the hint when you didn't see a bucket or a cooler or a gutting knife or any other fishy-type paraphernalia?"

He sighed with mock agony. "So what's for dinner, then?"

"You pick. Any restaurant in Dogwood."

"Main Street Seafood. I'm having fish for dinner tonight whether you like it or not."

"Should have seen that coming."

He chuckled. "You crack me up, Miriam. You're full of surprises."

"Surprises?" She cocked an eyebrow. "What do you mean?"

"What do I mean? Come on, Miriam. You're always so tough and cynical at work. Yet, you don't have the heart to kill a fish."

She shrugged. "I'm weird like that, I guess." She laughed. Then added, "But tell anyone, and you'll pay dearly. My little secret slips out, and so will yours, Bradley Fishpants, Navy hero who nobly fed the masses with your trousers."

Brad groaned. "That's blackmail."

"No it's not. It's a promise."

He tried to look smug, but couldn't help but laugh. "I haven't told many other people about my Fishpants story. Not even Sue."

There was a brief pause as Miriam thought about what to say next, now that Sue had been tossed into the conversation.

"So tell me again… what did Sue move to Croatia to do?"

"She went to work with orphans. They're rebuilding an orphanage and she's also going to be teaching and helping out with adoptions."

Miriam looked impressed. "That's very selfless, to walk away from her entire life here in Dogwood and go do something like that."

"I guess," Brad nodded. "And I guess it's probably pretty selfish of me to wish she hadn't gone."

"I'm sure it wasn't an easy decision for her to make."

"I don't know. She said she was really sad to leave me, but she seemed really excited about it, like she's been waiting all her life to do something like this. I just don't understand why she had to go so far to do it."

"Well, that's where the kids are."

"Yeah, but surely there are orphans here she could have helped."

Miriam waited for a second. Then she turned to Brad with a huge smile on her face. "Well, now that you mention it, there are. In fact, there are some orphans really closeby that I'd like you to meet."

Brad winced. "That's more in Sue's ballpark," he said. "I'm not much of a kid person."

"Oh, you have nothing to worry about," Miriam said. "Since catch-and-release isn't your idea of fun, let's go meet the orphans."

"Hey, catch-and-release is just fine with me," Brad protested. "I'm really not much of a kid person."

"Hey, this is my dream date, so I call the shots." She handed him one of the oars and flashed a smile. "Start paddling, Fishpants."

***

Miriam slowed the speed of her truck and made a quick turn down a dirt road.

Brad looked at his surroundings curiously. "Miriam, you're scaring me. Where are we going?"

But just as the words left his mouth, Brad found the answer to his own question. At the end of the dirt road was a small brick building, with a large fenced lot adjacent to it. Several dogs were running around inside the fence. A sign was mounted just in front of the brick building. As they came closer, the wording became clearer.

"Dogwood Humane Society," Brad read the sign aloud.

Miriam parked the truck and jumped out, waving her hand at Brad to follow.

Brad peered into the fence as they approached the door. "So these are the orphans, huh?"

"Yes. I never said they were kids. Never even said they were human."

"So what are we doing here?"

Miriam held the door open and motioned for Brad to come inside. "This is a small, privately owned animal shelter. It runs solely on donated money, manpower, and supplies. I volunteer sometimes. I just thought I'd look at the shelter's wish list and see what they need this week. I always try to bring a few things with me whenever I come in. A bag of dog food or kitty litter here and there really helps them out."

"Oh," Brad said, following Miriam inside. "I didn't know that you do this, Miriam."

"Well, it's only been a few months. I've always loved animals and I'd been wanting to volunteer with the Humane Society for years, but I didn't have the time until Homer passed away."

Inside the shelter, a chorus of dogs barked loudly from behind a closed door. Miriam greeted the attendant on duty and picked up a clipboard at the reception desk. "Dog food, cat food, bleach, paper towels, kitty litter… and they're running low on towels and blankets. Did you catch all of that, Fishpants?"

"Huh?" Brad asked. "Sorry, I was distracted. How many dogs are behind that door, anyway?"

"Close to twenty," the shelter attendant jumped into the conversation. "We're at maximum capacity right now."

Miriam made some notes on the wish list, checking off the items she was willing to donate.

Sad, isn't it?" Miriam said. "All those poor dogs, without homes. And cats, too."

"Twelve cats right now," the shelter attendant nodded. "One is a mama cat with a litter of five."

"I'm allergic to cats," Brad said.

Miriam looked up from the clipboard. "I hadn't pegged you for a cat person anyway, Fishpants. How about those dogs?"

Brad arched an eyebrow. "Oh, you don't mean... Miriam, I don't want to adopt a dog right now."

"Who said anything about adopting? Let's just go take a look at them and play with them for a little while, give them some attention."

He looked nervously at the door separating the reception office from the kennel. "Maybe another day," he said.

"Oh, as if you had a choice. This is my dream date, remember? You're still mine until the day is over." Miriam linked her arm through his and tugged him alongside her, into the kennel area.

Brad shuddered at the sight that awaited him. Chain link fencing runs separated what seemed like endless rows of dogs of all colors and shapes and sizes. Some of the dogs were on all four paws, barking loudly at the visitors, while some were curled up on a corner on the cement floor, looking sad, lost, and lonely. The fluorescent light bulb overhead was half burned out, and the half that was working buzzed loudly. "This is like... jail," Brad said. A chill passed through his body. "Poor dogs."

"How would you know? Ever been to jail?" Miriam poked a few fingers between the chain links of one of the kennels, stroking a German Shepherd's muzzle. He responded by licking her hand and wagging his tail with gratitude.

"Not as a prisoner," Brad said. "When I was a paramedic, we would occasionally get calls at the prison, and we'd have to treat and transport inmates. I didn't know what kind of crimes our patients had committed, but I still felt sorry for them, living behind bars and cinder block walls."

"Well, welcome to dog jail," Miriam said, reaching down to pet a small, mixed-breed dog in another run. "These poor guys' only crime is that they're homeless."

Brad looked around, frowning. He felt overwhelmed.

"Go ahead, Brad," Miriam said softly. "You can walk around. Take a look. Talk to them. If you'd like to take one out and go outside for a walk, just let me know. They're happy to have the company."

Brad nodded and began to walk down the narrow corridor separating the kennels on his left and right sides. "We had a dog when I was a kid," he said dreamily. "His name was Cupcake, and he was some kind of a terrier mix. He was more of my mom's dog, actually."

"I bet he was. Can't see someone like you giving a name like 'Cupcake' to a dog."

"He was a great little dog, though. I had a lot of fun with him."

Miriam followed on his heels as he walked the length of the kennel. "So that's the only dog you ever had?"

"Yeah."

"Ever thought about getting another one?"

Brad shrugged. "I've thought about it, yeah,"

"So... why not?"

"Sue's not a big fan of pets."

"Arooooo!" howled a cute mixed-breed dog as Miriam and Brad approached. Brad laughed, then kneeled down, putting himself face to face with the dog. The mutt stood up and crossed the run toward Brad.

"That's Scooter," Miriam said. She slid an index card out of a holder on the front of the dog's kennel and read it aloud. "Labrador-Beagle cross, approximately four years old, spayed and heartworm and parasite negative. She's been here for two weeks. Very sweet and friendly little girl. Ninety-five dollar adoption fee. Not a bad deal, huh, Fishpants?" She flashed him a used car-salesman-type grin, and wiggled her eyebrows playfully.

"Why is she here?"

Miriam went back to the cards, searching for the information. "Reason for intake: Owner surrender."

"That's all it says?"

"Yeah. Scooter belonged to someone else who either didn't want her or couldn't take care of her anymore, so she ended up here. In dog jail. Poor baby."

Brad poked his fingers through the fencing to touch the dog.

"Let her sniff you first," Miriam said.

As if on cue, Scooter sniffed Brad's hand and wagged her tail. Then she lowered her head and allowed Brad to touch her. He scratched her between her ears. A smile slowly spread across his face.

"Rooorooo," she murmured with delight.

"So what do you know about her?" Brad asked.

"She's a sweet girl. Not very high-energy, like most Beagles and Labs are. I suspect she's got something else mixed in with her, but not sure what it is. She eats, she sleeps, she poops and she drools a lot. That's about it."

"If I had a choice, that's all I'd do, myself."

"Sounds like the perfect dog for you, then." Miriam bent down and touched Scooter's floppy ears through the fencing. "She's also very loving. And loyal."

"She's… really sweet," Brad said. "And if I was in the market for a dog, I'd be interested. But I really shouldn't get a pet right now, Miriam."

"Why don't you take her for a walk?"

"I guess I can," Brad said. "But, just so you know, I'm not taking her home. I can't."

"Sure thing, Fishpants. Just get her out of that cage for a little while and let her get some exercise and sunshine. And that will be your good deed for the day." She opened the door to the kennel and snapped a leash onto Scooter's collar. "Take her out the back door and walk her around inside the fence for a little while."

"Okay."

Miriam saw Brad and Scooter out the door, then returned to the reception desk.

"How's it going with your friend?" The attendant asked.

"He's not ready for a dog just yet," Miriam said. "But he will be. Soon."

***

When Miriam dropped Brad off at his apartment, she was grinning from ear to ear. "Thank you for the dream date," she said. "I'd say that's the best fifteen thousand dollars I ever spent."

"Glad it was worth it," Brad laughed.

"I mean it," Miriam said. "I really did have fun with you today."

"I did too," Brad said. "In fact, I think we should get together again. A few more fishing sessions with you, and I'm quite certain I'd never have to use my fishpants method ever again."

They laughed. "You've got a lot of heart, Brad. I'll take you up on that sometime if you mean it."

"Of course I do. Now that I'm on my own again, my weekends are wide open. Just say when."

"Sounds good to me."

"Thanks, Miriam." He opened the door and put one foot on the ground to exit the truck. "And thanks for the trip to the shelter, too. I'm really glad we went."

She smiled. "I am too."

"I just hope you understand what I was trying to say back at the shelter. I never thought about getting a dog when Sue was here, because she didn't want a pet. Now that she's gone, if I bring a dog home, that means she's really gone, and she's not coming back. And that's a really big deal."

Miriam nodded. "I get it. Adopting a dog means you're letting Sue go."

Brad looked sad. "I really don't know if I'm ready," he said.

"I didn't mean to put any pressure on you."

"You didn't. I may get a pet one of these days. I just need some time."

"Well, whenever you're ready, you know where the Humane Society is."

Brad stepped out of the truck and motioned for Miriam to wait as he jogged around to the driver's side and opened the door. He reached inside the vehicle and wrapped his arms tightly around her in a bear hug, taking her by surprise. "Thanks for the dream date," he said.

Hugging him back, Miriam laughed. "I hope you know… I love you to pieces, Brad. And I'm here for you any time you need a friend. Or a sugar mama to bail you out from having to go on a date with Cassandra Putnam."

He laughed. "It goes both ways, Miriam. The friend part, I mean."

"Yeah, I got it."

"See you tomorrow at work, sugar mama," Brad said, waving to Miriam as he made his way to his apartment door.

"Sleep tight tonight, Fishpants!"

Chapter 8
Monday

It normally took Mel ten minutes to drive to work.

Not this morning. When Mel reached the main road that led her to the hospital, traffic was backed up for as far as the eye could see. She guessed it was because of a wreck.

After spending twenty minutes creeping along at a snail's pace, with a mile and a half still to go, she reached for her cell phone and called Donna.

"Med-Surg South, this is Donna." The normally cheery voice sounded frazzled and distraught.

"Hi Donna. Mel here. Just wanted to let you know I'm running late. It's not my fault, though. I'm stuck in traffic. It's bumper to bumper. I've never seen traffic like this in Dogwood before." The driver of the car behind her blared down on the horn, and as if on cue, every other driver on the road honked their horns in response. "You hear that?" She asked.

Donna chuckled. "Take your time," she said. "And get used to the chaos. There's plenty more of it waiting here for you."

"Huh?" Mel asked. "What's going on?"

"I'll save the surprise for when you arrive. I'll tell you this much now. When you start getting closer to the hospital, there will be police officers on the street checking for employee ID badges. Once you show yours, they'll wave you through to the parking deck and you'll be out of all the traffic congestion. But when you get parked, you'll have to fight your way into the building on foot. There are going to be reporters everywhere. If any of them ask you anything, just respond, "No comment" or "I'm not at liberty to make a statement" and that should get them off your back."

The car in front of her moved ahead about five feet, so Mel did the same.

"Donna, you've got me worried. What the heck is going on?"

"I would tell you, Mel, but there's a reporter hovering in the hallway just outside of my office. Trust me, you'll find out soon enough."

"Is everything okay? Has something bad happened?"

"Everything's fine. Don't worry. Just get here safely."

"Okay. See you when I get there." She hung up and turned on the radio, hoping that she could find a local newscast to give her a clue. After scanning through all of the local stations twice and finding nothing except for commercials for cell phones and attorneys, a lady reading the county's school lunch menu for the week, and 80's songs, she gave up and turned it off to retreat into silence.

***

Nearly forty-five minutes later, she reached the police officers' checkpoint that Donna had mentioned. She rolled her window down to let them examine her hospital badge. Satisfied, they waved her through. Mel parked on the top deck, claiming one of the three last spaces that she could see, and made her way down the long stairwell and out of the parking deck.

As soon as she crossed the street and found the footpath to the hospital's main entrance, Donna's second forewarning suddenly made sense, as reporters rushed to meet her. There were at least half a dozen of them. All were toting microphones, and were followed by cameras with blinding lights that blurred out the faces of the people hauling them around.

"Are you an employee of the hospital?" Two of them asked at the same time, almost in perfect unison.

"Yea—I mean, no comment," Mel quickly corrected herself.

It didn't discourage any of them, however. She imagined that her blue scrubs and the employee badge pinned to her chest answered the question for her. They proceeded with a new line of questions, in rapid-fire succession.

"Can you make any comment about his condition?"

"Do you know when he'll be discharged?"

"Can you tell us how this will impact the filming schedule?"

Mel glanced at the crowd that had formed a horseshoe around her, following her swift steps as she made her way to the entrance of the hospital. "Who are you talking about?" She finally asked.

"Devin Ryan," one of the reporters quickly responded.

Mel suddenly stopped. The entourage around her stopped with her, hoping that it was a sign that she would have some kind of comment to share.

"Really?" She asked in disbelief.

"We'd like to know about his condition," one of the reporters remarked. "Why don't you find out what's going on and come back and talk to us? You'll have an exclusive interview and you'll get to be on TV."

Mel narrowed her eyes. "No comment," she said.

"Anything you could tell us… anything at all… we'd like to know," another one hounded.

She whirled around and faced them. "I'm not at liberty to make a comment," she said curtly. But just as she finished her words, they spied a physician exiting his truck from the doctor's parking lot and tore across the lawn to reach him.

"Better him than me," Mel laughed to herself, as she entered the hospital and stepped into the elevator.

Devin Ryan. What in the world could have happened to Devin Ryan? She wondered. And what unit is he on?

When the doors opened, her question was answered.

Haylie and Brad rushed to greet her. Each of them took one of her arms and led her to the nurse's station.

"Mel," Brad began, "You're never going to believe this…."

"It's Devin Ryan," Haylie said excitedly. "He's here. Bed 3-B.

He was in a car wreck while they were filming a stunt yesterday. Can you believe it? We've got a movie star for a patient!" Haylie practically bounced up and down as she walked. Her long blonde hair, pulled back into a ponytail, swung from side to side like a pendulum.

Mel smiled smugly. "I saw the news on Saturday night. The movie crew has only been in town since Saturday, and already, the jerk went and got himself hurt."

Behind the nurse's station, Donna and Miriam broke free from a private conversation and looked up when Mel arrived.

"Glad you made it," Donna said.

"I got here as quickly as I could," she insisted. "I'm sorry it took me this long."

"It's okay," Donna assured her. "I know it's not your fault. But now that you're here, I need you. Got a big job for you."

"What's that?" Mel asked curiously. "Do I need to stand watch and fend off reporters?" She laughed softly.

"Not exactly," Donna replied. "I'm assigning you to be his nurse."

Mel stood up straight. Brad and Haylie must have felt the weight of the surprise pass through her body. They instantly released their grip on her arms, as if they had been shocked.

"What?" Mel asked. "Why me?"

Donna pulled her close and spoke in a low voice. "Here's the deal, Mel. Mr. Ryan was brought in by ambulance last night. Apparently, they were filming one of the movie scenes, which involved a car crash, and something went wrong. Either his seat belt failed, or else he just wasn't wearing it to begin with. He smashed into the steering wheel, so he's got several broken ribs, a collapsed lung, and a cardiac contusion that's causing some irregular heartbeats. Add an open fracture of the femur in his right leg to that, and you've got one banged up movie star. Anyway, he went into the O.R. around three o'clock this morning and after about six hours of surgery, he's in stable condition. He's got a chest tube in now and he's on a cardiac monitor, and lots of morphine, obviously."

Mel nodded as she listened, but her face was lacking her usual expression of empathy.

"Anyway," Donna continued, "You're the nurse on this unit that has the most experience with cardiopulmonary patients, so I want you to be Devin's nurse. We'll be doing frequent 12-lead EKG's on him and keeping an eye on those arrhythmias."

Mel looked surprised. "Donna, I worked for four years on the cardiac step-down unit. That doesn't necessarily mean that I'm the most qualified person to take care of him."

Donna raised one eyebrow. "I think it does," she said. "Do you have any objection to being Mr. Ryan's nurse?"

She bit her lip. "No," she said. "I'll give him the same care I would any other patient. I'm just a little bit freaked out about all of these reporters, and the publicity. I don't want anyone hovering over me and asking questions, like they did this morning when I was coming in to work."

"They won't," Donna said. "Mr. Ryan's publicist is here, and there's one reporter wandering the unit. Apparently he's someone that has a tight relationship with Mr. Ryan and was allowed to be here. But I will make sure that you don't have to worry about any of that. Your job is to take care of your patient. I'll be the point of contact for the press. Don't worry about anything else."

Mel thought for a minute, then relented. "Okay," she said. "If you really think I'm the best person to take care of him, and if you'll handle all of the press stuff, then fine, I'll do this."

Donna smiled. "Good," she said. "Go introduce yourself to him, then."

"I'll introduce you," Haylie offered, as she gripped Mel's arm once again and pulled her away.

"Haylie, I can do this myself," Mel whispered.

"Oh, I know you can. I just wanted another excuse to go in his room," she giggled. "He's soooooooo hot, Mel. HOT! He's just gorgeous! Even more handsome in person than in the movies." Haylie giggled excitedly and her ponytail spun again as she bounced up and down.

Mel sighed and shook her head. "If you say so."

"He's nice, too, Mel! I thought that all movie stars would be needy and demanding. But he's not. He's really sweet."

"How much time have you spent with him, anyway?"

"Only an hour or so," Haylie said.

Mel looked at her. "Really? How were you able to get into work so early?"

Haylie beamed. "I walked from home," she said.

Mel's eyes grew wide. "You're kidding."

"Nope. Didn't you hear the news the other day? I just moved to Dogwood Park Apartments. I don't even have to drive to get to work anymore." Haylie said proudly.

Smiling, Mel patted her on the shoulder. "Haylie, that's great! Congratulations!"

"Thanks!" Haylie said excitedly. "Let's go meet your patient." She pulled Mel into Devin Ryan's room.

Bed 3-A was vacant, and Mel guessed that it would stay that way because of Devin Ryan's star status. The lights and television were off, and the blinds were closed. It was quiet, and all that Mel could hear was the sound of the patient taking long, deep breaths. He was asleep.

"I don't want to wake him," Mel whispered.

"It's okay," Haylie whispered back. "He won't mind. I promise."

As they approached the side of his bed, Mel squinted her eyes in the darkness to better see him.

Devin Ryan was indeed sleeping on his back, with the covers drawn to his waist and his arms resting by his side. An IV had been placed in his right arm.

Haylie's right, Mel thought to herself. *He's a looker.*

In spite of the fact that he had suffered a traumatic injury and had endured surgery only hours before, Devin Ryan was indeed handsome, by any definition. His eyes were closed and his face was shrouded with the peace of sleep, but still, it was a handsome face. Tanned, with strong cheekbones and jaw lines, and big, handsome lips that formed his million-dollar smile during the waking hours.

His sandy-blonde hair was a bit tousled, but was still holding on to the style that his makeup and hair designers had meticulously created hours before. A slight shadow of a dark beard and moustache was beginning to form on his jaw and cheeks, and between his lips and nose.

He had no gown, only a bare chest with fresh surgical wounds and a tube that Mel was certain must be painful.

He looked so young and so fragile.

"How old is he, anyway?"

"Thirty eight," Haylie replied.

"Two years younger than I am," Mel mused, "but doesn't look a day over twenty-five."

Haylie touched his shoulder, and his eyes immediately opened.

"Hi Haylie," he murmured, fighting his way back from the haze of a sedative-induced sleep.

"Hi Devin," she said. "I want to introduce you to someone. This is Mel. She's a great nurse and she's going to take excellent care of you."

Devin's eyes wandered to Mel's face. He smiled. "Hi," he murmured.

"Hello Mr. Ryan," she responded.

"Devin," he corrected her. "None of that mister stuff in here. I'm too young to be a mister."

Haylie winked at Mel as she made her way out of the room.

Mel began again. "How are you feeling this morning?"

"Like hell," he responded, without missing a beat.

Mel nodded. "I bet you do. I hear that you had a pretty intense night."

His eyes widened. "That would be the understatement of the year,"

"Yeah. But I also heard that you're in stable condition now, and that you'll most likely bounce back from this just fine. Until the next time, right?"

"Next time?"

"Well, doing movie stunts is your career, isn't it?"

"Yeah. Why?"

"I watch celebrity news and read the tabloids from time to time. I know this isn't the first time you've been hurt. I don't get it. Why would you keep doing this to yourself? Getting all banged up for the sake of fame and fortune? Is it really worth it?"

He looked at her curiously. "Ouch," he said. "I take it you're not a fan."

"Definitely not a fan," she shot back. "The world we live in is violent enough, and people get hurt every day in real life. I don't see the point in bombarding ourselves with artificial images of it on TV and in the movies." She stared down at him smugly.

He smiled. "It's kind of nice to hear you say that."

"Huh?" She asked, deeply confused.

"It was very honest," he said. "And I respect honesty. Up until this point, everyone that's been in this room has done nothing but pay me compliments and ask for autographs and spout out catch phrases from my speaking lines in movies that were so stupid, even I don't remember them."

Mel crossed her arms and rocked back on her heels. "So if the movies were stupid, why did you make them in the first place?"

"Oh, I didn't know at the time that they were going to be stupid. I was just a young actor, doing the best that I could. Some of my earlier films were downright shameful. With horrible plots, unbelievable characters, there are some that I wish I could just buy up all the copies of and burn so that no one would ever see them again. Thankfully, I've got an agent now that does a much better job of reading scripts. He weeds out the stupid movies before they ever make their way to me."

"I personally think they're all stupid. I hear you do your own stunts. How much more stupid can you get? You could have stunt doubles if you wanted. People would stand in line for miles to get brutalized for you on film, but no, you insist on doing your stunts and putting yourself in harm's way."

He shrugged. "Guess that's my own little attempt at integrity."

"Very decent of you to include the word 'attempt' in that sentence. I see you really do appreciate honesty."

He wrinkled his brow. "Ouch again. Are you this nice to all your patients?"

"Nope. I'm going the extra mile for you. Can't you tell how bedazzled I am to have a celebrity on the unit?"

He grinned. "I wouldn't expect such sarcasm from such a pretty woman. What's got you so jaded?"

"At the moment, you," Mel retorted. "Let me be straight with you. I'm a good nurse and I'll take excellent care of you. But don't think for a minute that you're going to get star treatment with me. I don't think you're anything special. You're a human being just like me and all my other patients. So save the James Bond-brand charm for all the young giggly nurses, like Haylie, that think you're a hotshot. It won't work on me."

He cupped his hand over his heart. "Ouch. You're brutal," he said. "I like you already." Mel spotted an arrhythmia on the cardiac monitor. It wasn't dangerous, but she checked his vitals anyway. Blood pressure was 134/72. Pulse ox was 98.

"Everything okay?" He asked.

"Everything's fine." Mel nodded. "I know I'm going to regret asking this, but is there anything I can do for you before I go?"

"Yeah," he responded. "Smile."

"What?"

"I want to see you smile."

"I don't think so," Mel said in a huff, as she spun around and left the room.

Haylie, who had been listening in from outside the door, stepped back inside and parked herself in the chair next to him.

"Sorry about that," she apologized. "Mel must be in a funk today. She's normally not so... mean." Haylie leaned forward, shamelessly batting her eyelashes. "If you like, I could talk to my boss, Donna, and see if she could switch me and Mel, so that I could be your nurse".

"No, please don't."

Haylie was taken aback. "Really? You want Mel to be your nurse?"

Devin Ryan stared over Haylie's shoulder and into the sunlight beaming through the window. "I think I'm in love with her," he said.

Chapter 9
Tuesday

Mel awoke to the smell of food. She pulled on her bathrobe, knotted it at the waist, and journeyed into the kitchen. Jenny was standing in front of the stove, flipping a soy sausage patty over in the skillet.

"Good morning," Mel said.

"Hi Mom," Jenny replied. "I'm really sorry about the other night. You're right, I shouldn't have said some of the things I said and I really crossed a line. I hope that a nice homecooked vegetarian breakfast can make up for it."

Mel leaned against the wall. "I'm sorry too. I know I've been really snappy and short lately. I've just had several tough days in a row. But I'm ready to put all the negativity behind me and start fresh this morning. So I'm apologizing too, and I appreciate the breakfast as a peace offering."

"You're welcome," Jenny said. Grabbing two potholders, she reached into the oven and pulled out a French toast casserole.

"Mmmmm," Mel murmured dreamily, as the smell of warm wheat bread and cinnamon hit her. She helped Jenny move the food to the breakfast nook, and then set the table for two.

"Want me to wake up Mikey?" Jenny asked.

"No, let him sleep in until his alarm wakes him up for school. More snoozing makes for a less cranky teenager."

Jenny laughed. "Guess you learned that lesson with me a time or two, right?"

"You could say that."

Jenny poured two glasses of orange juice. They said grace and began to eat.

"It doesn't seem like that long ago that you were the moody teenager, and Michael was my sweet little boy," Mel began. "You both grew up so fast. How did that happen?"

"No clue. If I knew how to slow down time, I'd do it. I can't believe I'm going to be giving birth in a few months."

"Neither can I. In fact, I'll call the education department at the hospital today and find out when the next prepared childbirth class is. We should probably go ahead and sign up now. And they have a prenatal yoga class, too. You may like that one. And speaking of prenatal appointments, we need to find you a doctor here and transfer your medical records from school." Mel prepared a mental checklist, touching her right index finger to the fingertips on her left hand as she counted out the numerous things that needed to be done.

"Hey, Mom, about all that... the baby stuff, I mean..."

"Yes? What about it?"

"I think it's great that you're getting this involved. But I'm the one having the baby, and I can do some of this stuff myself, you know."

Mel looked away sheepishly. "So in other words, 'back off, Mom,' is what you're saying."

"Well... yes and no," Jenny smiled. "I want you to be my labor coach, and I want you to go to doctor's appointments and classes with me, but I don't want you to be worrying about me and the baby twenty-four seven and feeling like you have to take care of me – of us."

"I'm not worried, and I know you can take care of yourself. I'm just trying to be supportive. But I'll back off if you want me to."

"Easier said than done, Mom. You're a control freak. Admit it."

Mel looked down ashamedly. "Busted. I know."

Jenny grinned. "I was thinking that maybe if you had something else going on in your life, it would... distract you from me and the baby, and you wouldn't be worrying obsessively about the two of us."

"Something like what?"

"Like a new man."

"I thought we had this conversation last night. Not interested."

"His name is Rodney. He's a Gemini, six feet tall, with blonde hair and blue eyes, holds a management position at work—"

"Jenny!" Mel interrupted her. "What did you do?"

"I went to an online dating website and set up an account for you. You're quite the hot potato, Mom. Once I added your picture, you got twelve emails from guys who want to go out with you. I picked out the best one. You're meeting him for dinner tonight."

Mel leaned forward, bracing her elbows on the table and cupping her face in her hands. "Please tell me you're kidding. You put my picture out there for all the world to see?"

"Not the whole world. Just a small pool of local, paid subscribers to the dating website. You've got dinner reservations tonight at eight o'clock at Bella Cucina, that swanky new Italian restaurant downtown."

"Is he supposed to pick me up? You didn't give him our address did you? He's a stranger, for crying out loud—"

"Of course I didn't give him our address! Give me a little credit. You're meeting him there."

"And how will I recognize him?"

Jenny stood up and took her mother by the arm, pulling her into the living room, where she turned on the computer and danced excitedly as it booted up. She double clicked on a photo icon on the desktop, bringing the image of Mel's blind date into full view. Jenny elbowed her mother softly in the side. "What did I tell you? He's cute, isn't he?"

"He's probably an axe murderer," Mel sighed.

"Already did a background check on him, and I couldn't find a single axe murder in his history. Other than a speeding ticket four years ago, this guy's a saint."

"He probably has the I.Q. of a cardboard box."

"Au contraire. His profile says he's got a college degree in Business Administration, and he's currently working on his M.B.A."

"M.B.A. candidate? Then he's probably a frugal cheapskate. I bet he'll order the most expensive thing on the menu and then leave me to pay the bill."

"Mom, would you quit it? He's smart, and successful, and best of all, he's adorable!"

Mel retreated to her bedroom.

Thanks a lot Jenny. She sunk into her bed, wondering why she had even bothered getting up that morning. And then another thought crossed her mind.

Why not? What could it hurt?

"Admit it!" Jenny cried from just outside of Mel's bedroom door.

Mel sighed deeply, then rose from the bed and opened her door. "Okay," She relented. "You win. He's cute. But when I get home from work today, I'm going to need your help finding something to wear."

***

When Donna's phone rang, she wondered who would be calling her office so early in the morning.

"Med-Surg South, this is Donna."

"Hi Mom," Darius responded.

Although she recognized his voice, the sound still seemed unfamiliar after all this time.

"Hello, son. Did you get a good night's sleep?"

I slept great. Being back in my old room is just like old times. The only thing that's missing is Sean in the top bunk."

"Well, Sean took the bottom bunk after... you know."

"Yeah. I guess a lot of things changed after I went to prison. When I saw Jeannie getting ready for school, I just couldn't believe how much taller she is now. I guess I didn't notice when I first came home. Or maybe she grew another few inches overnight. Do you think that's possible, Mom?"

Donna smiled. "Never know," she replied. "Or maybe she's just so happy to have her big brother back that she's walking a little bit taller now."

"Well, one way or the other, she's all grown up. I can hardly believe it. Of course, that's not the only thing that's changed around here."

"What else have you noticed?" Donna asked.

"Well, um… the remote, for one," he said. "Looks like you guys got cable or satellite TV or something like that while I was gone. I tried to turn it on this morning but couldn't find anything but static."

Laughing, Donna shook her head. "I'll give you the TV-and-remote orientation when I get home," she said. "I hope you don't plan on spending too much time watching TV though. You need to get out and find yourself a job."

"I'm one step ahead of you. Ironing my shirt right now as we speak."

Good boy, Donna thought.

"Why don't you come by the hospital?" She asked. "I can introduce you to my co-workers, and we can go to lunch together in the cafeteria. And then I can take you to the human resources department to apply for some jobs here."

"Like what kind of jobs?"

"There are lots of jobs open right now. Food and Nutrition Services always needs people. Plus, I know that someone recently retired from Warehouse and Medical Supply, and they haven't filled his position yet. There are lots of possibilities here, Darius."

"That sounds good to me, Mama."

She paused for a minute. "Now you know that whatever kind of job you may get, you'll have to work hard, and you probably won't be making a lot of money at first. But you have to start somewhere. You realize that, don't you?"

"Yes ma'am."

"And you realize, if you get a job here, our schedules may not match up, so we may not be able to ride together, and you'd need to take the bus to and from work. I expect it to be a while before you can save up enough to buy a car."

"That's okay. I've got no problem with riding the bus."

She paused again. "Who are you and what have you done with my son?"

He laughed. "Come on, Mama. Give me some credit. I keep telling you, I've done a lot of changing."

Donna had been expecting a protest from Darius, and had already prepared a stern lecture for him about how he couldn't afford to be too proud to work hard at a job that paid modestly, but offered an honest living. When no such resistance came, Donna found herself speechless.

She reached for the picture that she kept on her desk of her children in their younger days. It had been taken just before Darius had dropped out of high school, and was the most recent portrait that she had of all three of them together. She focused on the handsome young man in the picture and remembered how much pressure had been put on him after his father had died. He had helped Donna care for his younger siblings, and even took on a part time job at a fast food restaurant after school three days a week to help with money.

He really had stepped up and tried his best to become the new man of the house. Donna wondered for a minute, as she had many times before, if she had failed him. If only she had been more insistent that he stay in school, or she had fought harder to find him a special tutor who could help him with his dyslexia, maybe he wouldn't have dropped out. If only she had lightened up on him at home and hadn't demanded so much of him, maybe he wouldn't have moved out. If only she had allowed him to finish his own childhood and had been more of a mother to him, maybe he wouldn't have ended up in prison.

She still believed that Darius was responsible for his own poor choices, but never stopped worrying that she was at least partly to blame. The least she could do, she realized, was to give him a second chance.

"I hope you know, I'm mighty proud of you, son," Donna said. "So why don't you come by my office around noon and we'll work on finding you a job. How does that sound?"

"Sounds good to me. I'll see you soon."

***

"Good morning, Ms. Benson," Brad said, sitting down in a chair and pulling it close to her bed. "Now what in the world are you doing snoozing in bed? You're supposed to be wearing your pink jacket and transporting patients to and from my unit, not getting admitted to it!"

Ms. Benson's eyes opened, and when she saw Brad, she smiled. "Hello there, my favorite nurse."

"Hello there."

"None of that Ms. Benson nonsense anymore, Brad. You can call me by my first name, Amena."

"Okay, Amena. That's a very pretty name."

"Why thank you," she said.

"It's very unusual. Is it foreign?"

"No, dear," she laughed. "I was the last of nine children. When my mother found out that she was expecting me, she prayed to God and said, 'Lord, let this be the last one!' And she decided that if I was a boy, my name would be 'Amen,' and if I was a girl, she would call me 'Amena' because it sounded a bit more feminine. Do you know why she chose 'Amen' for a name?"

"No ma'am."

"That's what you say when you finish a prayer. It means 'Let it be so' because you're at the end!" She laughed.

Brad chuckled as he checked her wristband, then watched as she swallowed her heart and thyroid medications. "So what happened to you?"

She shook her head slightly. "I guess I picked up a bug at the Dogwood Ball. I came home that night and didn't feel well, and was doing a lot of coughing and having trouble breathing. I was feeling feverish and wasn't able to eat or drink much. I felt faint yesterday, so I called 911. In the Emergency Department, they told me that I have pneumonia. That's some nasty stuff, dear. You need to wash your hands really good when you're done in here."

He nodded. "I certainly will. And you know I'll take good care of you, don't you?"

"The best care I could get anywhere on earth," Amena said, followed by a deep, raspy cough. Brad reached for a sputum basin and helped her lean forward as she spit out mucus streaked with blood. They both saw it and exchanged worried glances.

"Were you spitting up blood in the Emergency Department yesterday?"

"No. I was coughing up a lot of stuff, but it was just snotty looking yellow and green stuff. No blood. Is that bad?"

"Well… it could be," Brad said. Amena had been volunteering at the hospital for long enough to know that blood coming from the inside out was never a good thing. "But let me call your doctor. I'll go do that right now, okay?"

She flashed a dentureless grin and Brad's heart broke as he realized how frail her face looked without her signature toothy smile. Her skin color didn't look great either.

"How are you feeling?"

"Oh, very sleepy, dear."

"Why don't you get some rest while I call your doctor. I'll be back soon."

As Brad made his way to the nurse's station, he began to feel a bit panicked about Amena's condition. But the panic was quickly replaced by sheer dread when he saw Cassandra Putnam jogging down the hall.

"Look who's here," Miriam announced, with a sarcastic note in her voice.

Donna, Haylie, Mel and Brad looked up from their charting work at the nurse's station and focused on the approaching guest.

"Oh great," Brad grumbled. "Guess she couldn't take 'no' for an answer at the Dogwood Ball."

Miriam laughed. "Oh, you think this is about you? I bet you anything she heard that Devin Ryan is on our floor, and she's come to slobber all over him."

"Not looking like that," Haylie said. "She looks like she just rolled out of bed on laundry day."

"That's enough," Donna snapped. "I don't care what she's here for. I expect all of you to treat her with courtesy and respect. If she does anything out of line, let me know, and I'll deal with it. Otherwise, you need to give her the same care and attention you would any other guest of our unit."

When Cassandra reached the nurses' station, she was out of breath. She was dressed in the uncharacteristically non-glamorous attire of blue jeans, a frumpy-looking tee shirt and tennis shoes. Her face was anguished.

"Excuse me," she pleaded, "I'm looking for my mother, Amena Benson."

All five of the nurses' eyes fixed on her.

Brad suddenly felt foolish, as did Miriam.

She's not here on a manhunt after all, Brad said to himself. *She's here for her mother, poor thing.* He quickly rose from his seat. "I'll take you to her." He motioned with his hand for her to follow him as he walked toward Amena's room.

After Brad and Cassandra were out of earshot, Miriam sighed. "Guess I was wrong."

"What's going on with her mother?" Haylie asked.

Donna tapped out a sequence of keystrokes on the computer, pulling up Ms. Benson's patient record. "She was brought to the Emergency Department via ambulance."

"When was she admitted?" Miriam asked.

"Yesterday. Second shift, after all of us had gone home." Donna continued reading. "Bless her heart," she murmured softly. "She's got pneumonia." She leaned closer to the computer screen. "Her WBC count is through the roof," she said.

"Brad is her nurse," Miriam said, as she glanced over at the dry-erase board listing patients and their assigned nurses. "He can tell us how she's doing when he gets back."

"I should have put two and two together when I saw them sitting together at the Dogwood Ball," said Mel. "I remember now that Ms. Benson was saying that she would bid on Brad, but that she was sure she'd get outbid by her daughter."

Miriam nodded. "I remember that too. How ironic. Brad's got both of them to deal with now."

"Ms. Benson just adores him," Haylie said. "She calls him her favorite nurse."

"I know," Mel said. "And he's pretty attached to her too. He's mentioned a couple of times that she reminds him a lot of his late grandmother. Very similar looks and the same sweet personality."

Donna looked at Mel. "Not to change the subject, but how is

Brad holding up? He hasn't said much about Sue leaving. Actually, he hasn't said much lately."

"I guess he's fine," Mel said.   "I'm sure he misses her, but he's hanging in there."

"I spent Sunday with him," Miriam interjected. "He talked a little bit about Sue. I think he's still in shock over the whole thing and he needs some time to adjust."

"He's not the only one," Mel said softly. She figured that everyone else would find out her news eventually, and now was as good a time as any to share it.

"What do you mean?" Haylie asked.

Mel looked at her three fellow nurses. "I've got some major drama going on in my life too," she said. "It's Jenny. She's pregnant."

Mel watched as all of their eyes grew large. Then they looked at each other, searching for the right words to say.

"Oh my," Donna offered. She looked at Mel sympathetically. "I guess I should be asking how you are holding up then?"

"Just peachy," she said, with more than a hint of sarcasm. "Would love to stick around and tell you more, but I've got to go check on Devin Ryan."

"Oh, do you need any help?" Haylie asked excitedly.

"Sorry to disappoint you, but no," Mel replied with a sigh, as she trudged into the patient's room and washed her hands.

***

"Good morning, Mr. Ryan," Mel said, pulling the privacy curtain aside.

"It's Devin," he said. "Mr. Ryan was my father."

Mel cocked an eyebrow. "Right. How are you feeling this morning?"

"Sore," he said. "Hurts when I breathe, hurts when I move, hurts when I talk…"

"Well you can fix that all very easily. Quit breathing, quit moving and quit talking."

"I can quit moving and talking, but the breathing part could be a problem. What do you suggest… artificial respiration? Are you qualified to do that?" His brow was wrinkled with mock worry.

"You're a funny man, Devin Ryan." Mel's words dripped sarcasm.

"You called me Devin," he said. An arrhythmia danced across the screen on the cardiac monitor.

She pressed a button to inflate his blood pressure cuff. "Don't get so excited. Your heart just went into a funky rhythm. If calling you by your first name does the trick, then maybe I should go back to calling you Mr. Ryan."

"I told you, my Dad was Mr. Ryan, not me."

"Was? As in, he's not Mr. Ryan anymore?"

"What I meant is that he died. Before I was born, actually. Never even met the guy."

"Sorry to hear that."

"It's okay. You can't miss what you never had."

Mel shrugged. "I don't know about that," she said. "Surely you feel something for your father, even though you never met him… don't you?"

"Well, I guess so. I think I miss the idea of him; of simply having a father, more than anything else. I've seen pictures of him, and I've heard stories about him from my mom and other family and friends, but that's as close as I've ever come to him."

Mel looked at his blood pressure reading. "Good blood pressure," she said. "124 over 69. That's pretty good considering all you've been through." She unwrapped her stethoscope from around her neck and checked his lung sounds. "Lungs sound good too."

Devin grinned. "Really? That almost sounded like a compliment."

"No," Mel shot back. "Simply stating a fact."

He rolled his face away from her, toward the window. "Should have known," he said. "My nurse hates me." He sniffled and pretended to cry.

Mel watched him for a minute, thinking that she should have been annoyed. Instead, she found herself fighting the urge to laugh.

"Waaaah," Devin wailed. "You can correct me at any time, you know." He paused for a minute, turned his head slightly to peek at her from the corner of his eye, and then turned his face away again. "WAAAAH!" He yelled.

At last, Mel giggled. Devin turned his head around quickly. "Finally," he said.

"Finally what?"

"A smile."

Mel quickly pinched her lips together, trying her best not to continue smiling. "Uh-uh," she protested.

Devin pushed a button, raising the head of his bed up slightly. His eyes were fixed on her. "Mel, do you really dislike me that much? If there's something that I said or did to offend you, I apologize."

Mel suddenly felt ashamed. She sank into a chair. "You haven't done anything wrong, Devin, and no, I don't dislike you. I just dislike... the idea of you."

He smiled slightly. Mel tried not to think about how handsome he was, now that he had some color back in his face, and a sparkle in his eyes.

"So what's your 'idea' of me?"

Mel shrugged. "I've watched your movies, and just like you said, a lot of them are just plain stupid."

"Can't argue with you," he offered. "But you know they're just movies, and the roles that I play aren't real. I make action movies because I love the stunts and the excitement. It's just an added bonus that I get paid for it."

She shook her head. "That's not really it," she said. "I guess it's just..."

He watched her, giving her a moment to collect her thoughts. She looked away as she struggled to find the right words.

"All the other times that you're on camera, in the news or on awards shows or even on the covers of tabloids... I just haven't seen any positive images of you. In fact, every time that I've ever seen you, it's been with a bottle of liquor in one hand, a cigarette in the other and a trashy looking girl half your age either at your side or on your lap."

Devin sat quietly. Mel wasn't sure what he would say. It wasn't like he could convince her that he'd never done any of those things. She'd seen proof with her own eyes too many times.

"I know it's wrong for me to judge you based on the last picture I saw of you on the cover of a tabloid," Mel resumed, "but I've looked at you in the magazines and on my TV and have never found anything appealing or classy about you."

Devin slowly nodded. "I can't argue with you, Mel. I definitely went through some wild spells in my career and I've done some things that, as you said, aren't very classy, and I'm not proud of them."

Mel sank back into the chair and crossed her arms. "You talk about it all as if it was in the past."

"Because it is," he said. "There are a lot of things about me that you wouldn't know based on what you've seen on TV or read in magazines."

"The camera never lies," Mel said.

"No, it doesn't. But what people don't realize about pictures and videos of celebrities acting stupid is that they never go away. In this wonderful age of digital media, anything you get caught doing on camera can stick around forever, and can resurface and come back to haunt you when you least expect it. If you've seen any pictures or videos of me recently in which I'm smoking, or drinking, or clinging onto younger women, they're at least a year old."

Mel looked at him skeptically. "You're saying you gave up your party boy ways?"

"Something like that. I'm a different person now."

"You don't have to explain to me," Mel said, looking away. "You don't need my approval."

"I'm not asking for it," he responded. "I'm just asking you to consider that whatever it is that you're holding against me, whatever it is that you think you know about me... it may be different from the person that I really am. The person I am now, anyway."

"I'm not holding anything against you, Devin."

"Your stethoscope was really cold and you held THAT against me," he said, playfully. "How about warming that thing up next time?"

She rose to leave the room. "Anything else I can do for you?"

"Smile," he said.

Mel turned and walked out of the room.

***

At the nurse's station, David Carl rested his elbows on the desk and chatted with Miriam, Haylie and Donna.

Mel was happy to see him, and jumped into the conversation. "David, hi! What brings you up to Med-Surg South today?"

"Hi Mel," he said, turning to her. "I came to visit one of the patients on Med-Surg North, and thought I'd stop by the South side to see how all of you are doing over here."

"Lots of people are stopping by these days, now that Devin Ryan is one of our patients," Haylie swooned. "Speaking of Devin, I'll still trade you, Mel. Mr. Crowell is back in bed 4-A. Want to swap?"

"Tempting," Mel said.

"How is Devin?" David asked.

"He's doing well," Mel said. "He's a jerk, but he's recovering nicely."

Donna arched an eyebrow. "That's not the kind of attitude you need to have toward your patients," Donna scolded.

"Well pardon me for being blunt, but he is," Mel vented.

"Maybe he's not a jerk," David said. "Maybe it's just a clash of personalities."

"Lucky me, I've got no jerks this shift," Brad bragged as he stepped around the corner and joined the group. "I've got Ms. Benson. She reminds me of my Grandma Lillian. Looks just like her, and every bit as sweet."

"Awww," said Donna. "That's adorable. You'll have to bring a picture of Grandma Lillian to work with you so you can show us."

"I'd have to dig for one," Braid said. "She died ten years ago."

Donna frowned. "Were you close to her?"

Brad nodded. "I sure was. I still miss her."

"Well it's no wonder you're attached to Mrs. Benson," Haylie mused. "It's like having your Grandma back, isn't it?"

"I don't know. Maybe. But I am worried about her."

"And I'm worried about Mr. Crowell too," Haylie said. "I know he's given us all a hard time, but I guess he can't help it. He's been hospitalized so much this past year, I can't imagine what it's like to be in his shoes."

"So what are all of you using as S.E.M.P.E.?"

The five nurses exchanged curious glances.

"I have no clue what you're talking about," Donna was brave enough to say. "Another acronym must mean more rules and regs. Don't tell me we've got to go through more task forces and surveys for something totally new…"

David chuckled. "Oh, no. It's nothing like that." He reached for a rubber glove and held it up on display. "You all are familiar with P.P.E., correct?"

"Personal protective equipment," Haylie said.

"Right. On any given day, this rubber glove could very well be the only thing standing between you and something really nasty, like a bloodborne pathogen. It will protect you from a lot of things, but there are some things that it won't protect you from."

"Like what?" Miriam asked.

David tossed the glove into the trash. "It will give you absolutely no protection from stress. Emotional attachment to your patients. Compassion fatigue. Loss and grief. You need S.E.M.P.E. for all of that."

"And again, we have no clue what that is." Miriam said in a huff.

"Spiritual, Emotional, and Mental Protective Equipment." David pointed his index finger with each word, as if pointing to the phrase on an imaginary screen. "Your job has lots of health hazards that go beyond just threats to your physical health. Your heart, your mind and your spirit are on the line too. You have to arm yourself with some kind of protection, to give yourself strength for dealing with the human side of health care."

Intrigued, each of the nurses leaned in a bit closer.

"So what do you recommend?" Mel asked.

"There are lots of things you can do," he began. "For starters, you need to get a full eight hours of sleep every twenty-four hour period. With you nurses, I know it can be hard. First shift, second shift, third shift, extra shifts… I know that day sometimes blurs into night, and yesterday somehow becomes today, and you find yourself getting very little sleep. Your mind and your body can't recuperate and recharge after a full day's work without those precious eight hours. How many of you get less than your full eight hours?"

Each of them looked away guiltily. "I know I haven't been sleeping great lately," Donna sighed. "Lots going on in my life right now. Big changes."

"Then you're coping with some loss," David said. "You're going through a grieving period."

Donna's eyebrows shot up with a look of curiosity. "No, no one has died or anything," she explained. "The major change in my life is actually a good one. I haven't lost anything."

"Death isn't the only form of loss," David said. "Every change in life is a loss. There's always the loss of the way things used to be. Changes in your life may be good, but there may be things about the adjustment that are challenging or uncomfortable. Maybe that's what's keeping you up at night?"

Nodding slowly, Donna sighed. "Maybe," she pondered. "That makes sense."

"Rest is essential," David said. "Not just physical rest, but emotional rest. You all need to take a day off every now and then. Anybody else guilty?"

Several fingers pointed at Mel.

"Hey," she said, defensively, "I'm picking up every extra shift that I can because I need the money."

"But I bet you're tired," David scolded. "And weary health care workers put their patients at risk. Lack of sleep in a health care environment is strongly tied to medical errors."

Mel felt embarrassed. "I just don't have much of a choice right now," she said, feeling a bit peeved that her friend would put her on the spot, knowing her circumstances.

"That's understandable," David said. "But you still need to escape every now and then. You need to take your breaks throughout the day, even if you've only got thirty seconds. You can go on break in your mind. In fact, we'll do it right now. All of you – right now – close your eyes."

As good pupils would do, they closed their eyes as instructed.

"Imagine a place that makes you feel safe or happy. Go there in your mind. Imagine the sights, and the smells, and the way that it feels to be there. Take a deep breath."

David watched the second hand on his watch. "Okay," he said softly, after thirty seconds had passed. "Come back to work now."

Everyone opened their eyes except for Miriam.

"Leave me alone, everyone," she said. "I'm at the spa getting a massage from a really hunky European guy named Hans."

Everyone laughed, including David. "Was the thirty second escape good for you?"

"Yes," Donna and Haylie said.

Brad shrugged. "No offense, but I'm not into this happy place stuff."

"His idea of a perfect escape is a cold beer and a video game with his friends," Mel said, giving him a playful nudge with her elbow.

"Nothing wrong with that," Miriam offered. "If that's what recharges his batteries, then so be it."

"I think you're right, Miriam," David nodded. "Brad's doing something very good, actually, in that he's spending some time with friends blowing off steam. It's really easy for nurses to become isolated, isn't it? You work long hours taking care of your patients – and each other – and then you go home and take care of your families. It seems like no matter where we turn, there are demands on our time and attention. Everyone needs to spend some time around people who can give something back to us, whether it's a pat on the back, or a kind word or just listening. Your friends can help you do that."

Haylie arched her eyebrows, deep in thought. "It's funny you'd say that," she interjected. "I made a new friend named Jaime from Med-Surg North, and I just moved into the same apartment complex as her. We're literally fifteen steps away from each other, but we haven't gotten together to hang out yet. It's my fault, really. She's invited me over to her apartment for dinner a couple of times, and I just haven't been able to find the time to go. I really want to, but like you said, David, I've got all of these other people to take care of, and at the end of the day, I'm exhausted."

"If you're too tired to get together for dinner, then why not a phone call or an email instead?" David suggested. "With a true friend, it doesn't have to be all or nothing. As long as you make contact with others and you've got someone that you can talk to and share things with, you're doing something good for yourself. You've got a caring connection – which is a very powerful weapon to include in your S.E.M.P.E. arsenal."

Donna laughed. "Arsenal... weapons... you make it sound like we're at war."

"Well, aren't you?" David asked, grinning. "You're fighting for your own mental, physical and spiritual health and well-being. You've got stress and strain coming at you from every angle as a nurse. Just because those things are unseen doesn't mean that they aren't taking a toll on you. The way I see it, you walk into combat every day."

"So this unit is essentially a combat zone," Brad said. "I can't argue with that. I've had more stressful days here than I ever did in the military."

"I'm not surprised," David agreed. "Did you ever go into combat while you were in the Navy?"

"No, thankfully."

"But you did combat simulations, didn't you?"

"Oh yeah. Plenty of those."

"And what did you do to protect yourself?"

"From what, the stress?"

"From the enemy. All of the bullets, the shrapnel, the explosives..?"

"Oh. We wore protective armor," he said. "Vests, helmets, stuff like that."

David smiled and pointed to each of them. "So where is your armor?" He asked, his eyes twinkling. "Not for your body, but for your mind? And your heart? And your morale and your spirit?"

The five nurses looked at each other.

"Well," said Donna, "I pray. All the time. The Bible says that we go into spiritual warfare, and I guess prayer would be our best armor for battles."

David looked at the rest of the nurses. "Do any of the rest of you pray?" He asked.

"Sometimes," Haylie shrugged. "But not the way the rest of you do. I'm Jewish, and don't pray to Jesus or Mary or anyone else but God. And I don't talk about my religion much, because we're in the 'Bible Belt' here, and people can be very judgmental if you don't believe the same things they do."

Donna looked wounded. "Well as you know, I'm an evangelical Christian, but I hope I've never made you feel judged... or uncomfortable, Haylie," Donna said.

"No, I wasn't talking about you, Donna," Haylie said. "I'm just speaking about people in general. Sometimes people will ask me what church I go to, and when I tell them that I'm Jewish and I go to synagogue, they give me this weird look, like I just told them I have an incurable disease or something."

"And I can relate," Miriam said. "I consider myself a Christian, but I'm not a church-goer. Sometimes I get dirty looks and strange questions from people because I choose not to. Or I get called a hypocrite or some variation of it. But I'm entitled to my own beliefs and can practice my faith however I want. I shouldn't have to explain myself to anyone."

"You're not alone, Miriam. I haven't been to church in a while either," Mel said. "But I still pray every day. Although I wonder sometimes if anyone's getting the message on the other end of the line. I've done a lot of praying lately, and haven't gotten a lot of answers."

Brad shook his head. "Sorry to keep being the problem child here, but I'm not a believer in prayer and God and all of the other-worldly stuff."

"And this is all okay," David said. "We're all different folks, and as Miriam said, we're entitled to have our own beliefs and our own faith, and we can worship or pray – or opt not to – if that is what we choose. But getting back to the question I asked you all a moment ago – do you pray? There's another part to that question. I next want to ask you. What is prayer?"

"Talking to God," Donna said.   "Giving praise.   Asking for forgiveness for the things that we've done wrong.   And asking for blessings."

"Okay," David said. "That's Donna's definition of prayer. Anyone else care to share one?"

The rest of the group was silent.

"Don't look at me," Brad laughed.   "Like I said, I'm not a religious person."

"It's okay. You don't have to be," David assured him. "Prayer means different things to different people."

Brad looked confused. "How's that?"

David pointed to a bookshelf behind the desk at the nurse's station. "There's a dictionary right behind you. Grab it for us, please."

Brad did as David requested, pulling the heavy hardcover book off of the shelf.

"Look up the word 'prayer.' See what it says."

Brad found the "P" tab on the side and opened the dictionary. He thumbed through several pages, finally locating the word. "Prayer," he said. "A petition to God. An act or practice of praying to God. Worship." He looked up and cocked an eyebrow, challenging David to explain how exactly this was not considered religious.

"Keep reading," David shot back with a smile.

Brad found his place in the book again. "A petition. A hope or chance."

"Ah." David's face lit up. "Hope. You don't have to be religious to have hope, do you?

"I guess not."

"So your prayer can be hope, just as the dictionary says. If you could hope for one thing right now... for yourself, and all of your patients, and all of your co-workers and all the rest of the world, what would it be?"

"Let me think." Brad's eyes wandered to the floor as he lost himself in deep thought. Not taking his assignment lightly, he took a quick inventory of the people in his life and what he would grant them, if he could pray it into existence.

Good health, maybe?

He visualized Mrs. Benson and Devin, and all of the other patients from Med-Surg South who were struggling with illnesses or were recovering from painful surgeries. If only he could take away their physical pain and bring healing, his prayer would be well spent.

But then he thought about Mel and her emotional pain. How she still came to work some days with eyes that were bloodshot and weary from crying. Physically, Mel was fit as a fiddle. Emotionally, she was hurting as much as any post-op patient on the unit.

If not health, what then? Happiness?

And then he thought about Sue. She'd been both healthy and happy. Yet, something restless within her had led her away from her home and her friends to serve a cause that she felt was worthwhile. What was it that she was searching for? And had she found it?

What next? Fulfillment?

He closed his eyes as he imagined her surrounded by orphaned children, like in the picture of her sister Sandra. She was smiling. Then, he could hear the children laugh, and he smelled the ash and soot of the orphanage that had burned down during the war.

"I know," he said at last. "Peace. I would wish for everyone to have peace."

Smiling, David nodded. "Okay then. So what will your prayer be? What is your hope?"

"Well, I hope for peace for the world, of course. But I also hope that I can help the person right in front of me to find it."

"So that can be your prayer," David suggested. "It's as simple as saying – or thinking – these words: 'May there be peace in the world, far and near, and may I bring peace to this person right here.' And there you have it."

Donna smiled. "I like that. It rhymes. Easy to remember."

"Do all of you wash in and wash out when you're going to take care of a patient?" David asked, referring to the practice of washing hands when entering a room, and washing hands before leaving a room.

Each of the five nurses nodded emphatically.

"Why not pray in and pray out? Hope in, hope out?" He posed the question. "Just like washing your hands, it can be part of your personal protection."

Brad closed the dictionary and placed it back on the shelf. "I'll be honest, it's just not my thing. Prayers, mantras, words of hope… whatever you want to call them… they're still just words to me. I don't really believe that they have the power to change anything."

David grinned. "Well let's do a little experiment, then. Stand up for me, will you, Brad?"

Brad stood, curious to know what David's next move would be.

"Hold out your dominant arm," he ordered. "Whichever hand you write with. Just hold it straight out from your body, extending all the way at the shoulder."

Brad stretched his left arm out. David stepped behind Brad, placing his right arm on Brad's left shoulder, and his left hand on Brad's wrist. The other nurses gathered closer to watch.

"Okay, Brad," David began. "You're a pretty strong guy, aren't you?"

Grinning, Brad nodded. "I suppose. I can bench two hundred pounds."

"So I want you to tell yourself that you're strong. Say it aloud, five times."

"I am strong," Brad said. "I am strong, I am strong, I am strong, I am strong."

"Good," David said. "Now I'm going to press down on your arm as hard as I can. I want you to resist. Don't let me push your arm down."

"Okay."

David pressed on Brad's arm. The veins on his forearms bulged as he resisted.

"Nice job," David said. "How did that feel? Was it pretty easy for you to resist?"

"Yeah. It took a little work, but you told me not to let you press my arm down, so I didn't."

"So you think you could do it a second time?"

"Sure," Brad said. "Go for it."

David pressed down on Brad's arm. Once again, he resisted, and Brad's arm didn't budge.

"One more time," said David. "Only this time, I want you to tell yourself something different. Instead of telling yourself you are strong, I want you to tell yourself you are weak. Five times, just like before."

Brad smirked. "Okay. I am weak. I am weak. I am weak, I am weak, I am weak."

"Ready?"

He nodded.

David pressed down on Brad's wrists. To the astonishment of everyone observing, Brad's arm dipped down to his side. He rocked back on his heels slightly, surprised to have been thrown off balance by the pressure against his arm.

"What the—?" Brad shook his arm as if it had gone to sleep.

"Oh my," Donna said. "Did you press harder, David?"

"Not at all. I actually had to use less pressure this time. Brad was weak. He told himself so. His body believed it, and reacted accordingly."

"Maybe his arm was just tired," Haylie suggested. "He resisted the pressure twice already, so maybe his muscles are fatigued."

"Well if that's the case, then he'll be too tired to resist a fourth time. What do you say, Brad, shall we try it?"

"Yeah," he said. "I'm freaked out now. I can't believe you moved my arm. I was trying to resist even harder, because I was determined to prove you wrong."

"Well let's get you strong again. Tell yourself that you're strong. Five times."

Brad nodded. "I am strong. I am strong. I am strong. I am strong. I am strong."

David pressed down on his arm, and Brad resisted with no problem.

"Amazing," Miriam said. "I want to try now!"

"Pair up with each other and give it a try," David suggested. Donna and Mel paired up, as did Haylie and Miriam. Each time, the results were the same. The nurses were mesmerized.

"Now do you think differently about the power of words?" David asked Brad.

"I'm certainly surprised," he said. "But yeah, I guess I do."

Haylie's eyes suddenly lit up. "I get it, David. S.E.M.P.E. It's a mnemonic," she said, smiling.

"A what?" Miriam asked.

"A mnemonic. It's a word you use to remember a list of things. S.E.M.P.E. means Stress, Emotional, and Mental Protective Equipment," Haylie said. "But it also stands for the list of protective equipment itself. "S" means sleep. "E" means escape. "M" means make contact with others. "P" means prayer... and hope."

David nodded. "You figured it out," he said. "But what about the last E? We didn't get there yet."

The five nurses looked at each other, each deep in thought and searching for the answer to David's impromptu quiz question.

"Exchange... Excel... Engage..." They mumbled ideas.

"Enjoy," David finally said, grinning from ear to ear. "If you can't find something every day to smile and laugh about, and feel thankful for, and just plain enjoy, then you're not really living." He paused for effect. "Life is happening right now as we speak. And this life that you've been given ... it's the only one you've got. No exchanges, no refunds, no starting over at the beginning if it doesn't go the way you planned. Happiness is a choice, and life is what you make of it."

"Amen to that," Donna said softly.

"And if you'll excuse me, I need to be on my way," David said.

"Come visit us again," Mel said.

"Oh, I will. I'll be back in a couple of days to see how all of you are doing with your S.E.M.P.E."

"Oh no," Haylie groaned playfully. "You mean we've got homework? I didn't even know we were in class," she laughed.

David grinned. "It will be the easiest homework you've ever had," he said. "You – call your friend Jaime back and take a few minutes to catch up with her. That's yours," he suggested.

"What about me?" Donna asked.

"Get some sleep, fearless leader. Your troops are counting on you."

"And me?" Mel piped in.

"A day off – if you can afford to take one. And if not, find other ways to escape. Or contact a friend."

Brad looked at David with a smirk. "Alright, I'll play along. I'll try the pray in, pray out," he said. "Let's see if my hope going out into the world will make a difference."

"What about me?" Miriam asked.

"Oh, that's easy. Close your eyes and finish getting your massage with Hans."

They all laughed.

***

Later that evening, Jenny covered Mel's eyes with her hands and led her to the full-length mirror in the hallway.

"I'm scared to see this," Mel confessed.

"Ta-dah!" Jenny shouted as she removed her hands from Mel's face.

At first glimpse in the full-length mirror, Mel cringed. Jenny had ironed her mother's hair straight with a ceramic iron, and had applied way too much makeup. She'd also dressed Mel in a short red skirt, black halter top, and high-heeled black leather boots. Large, loopy earrings dangled from Mel's ears and a black choker necklace was firmly fastened around her neck.

"Well... what do you think?" Jenny asked.

"I think I look like a really old hooker," Mel sighed. "Just give me a feather boa and a lit cigarette, and that should complete the look."

"Oh mom, stop," Jenny protested. "You look amazing. You look ten years younger. No... twenty! You look twenty years younger."

Shaking her head, Mel proceeded to remove all traces of Jenny's makeover, starting with the boots and working her way up to the earrings. "Just because I still wear the same size as you doesn't mean that I should borrow your clothes. I don't want to look twenty years younger, Jen. Or even ten." Mel thought about Cassandra Putnam squeezed into the high school prom dress at the Dogwood Ball, and a chill passed through her body. "I don't want to be one of those old women who shops in the juniors store, just because I can wear juniors sizes."

"You're only as old as you feel," Jenny pouted. "I personally think you look great in my clothes." Jenny fished the red skirt off of the floor and slipped it on over her shorts. She struggled to button it.

"It might help if you take your shorts off first," Mel said.

"No, it's not that," she reflected. "I'm getting a belly."

Jenny butted in front of Mel and turned to the side, staring at the reflection of her own profile in the mirror. Indeed, Mel could see a bump in Jenny's belly.

For a long moment, silence filled the space between them.

"I still sort of can't believe this is happening to me," Jenny said. Then she reached into her pocket and pulled out a small square of paper. She handed it to her mother. "I went to the doctor today while you were at work," she said. "And they did my first ultrasound."

Mel's heart skipped a beat as she looked at the image of her grandchild. The sonographer had captured a perfect view of the tiny, round face. The baby was sucking on its thumb.

"Oh," Mel gasped. "Beautiful."

"You think so? Michael says the baby looks like Spider Man."

Mel laughed. "Is it a boy or a girl?"

"We couldn't get a clear view of the baby's genitals, so we don't know just yet." Jenny said. "Although I just have this feeling that it's going to be a boy. Dad says he would love to have a grandson."

Mel looked up from the ultrasound picture and shot Jenny a wounded look.

"I'm sorry I didn't tell you first," Jenny said.

"It's okay. I understand why. And... I'm glad that your Dad is being supportive."

"Thanks." Jenny sighed. "This seems kind of wacky, doesn't it?"

"What seems wacky?"

"You're getting ready to go out on a date, and I'm the one at home getting ready to have a baby."

"Wacky would be a good word," Mel said. "Speaking of going out on my date, I can't go in a slip and panty hose."

Jenny knelt down to pick up the rest of her clothes off the floor. "Guess we'd better find you something else to wear since these duds don't make the cut."

"I don't mean to hurt your feelings. I just think I'd be a lot more comfortable wearing something from my own closet."

"It's okay. I'm getting quite comfortable with rejection."

"What do you mean by that?"

Jenny looked down at the floor. "I've called Jeremy a few times and he's not calling back."

"Well... maybe he's just busy, honey."

Jenny looked as if she might cry. "You know when I said that we talked about getting married and we both decided that it wasn't right for us?"

"Yes..."

"We did, but it was more like me talking about marriage, and him deciding that it wasn't right for us."

"Oh... honey..."

"I don't think he's going to be much of a father," Jenny said, beginning to sniffle. "I think I'm in this alone, Mom."

"No you're not." Mel wrapped an arm around her. "I don't think you're going to get the American Dream package with this baby, complete with the perfect husband and white picket fence, but you'll always have a home with me, and you'll never be alone. Instead of focusing on what you don't have, count your blessings and give thanks for what you do have. Don't get all upset. It's not good for a pregnant woman."

Jenny melted into her mother's arms, weeping uncontrollably.

"I need you to stay strong, kiddo. My little grandbaby needs you to cheer up and think good thoughts to help it grow up strong and healthy."

Jenny sighed. "I know, Mom. It's just hard to do when things aren't going my way."

"Happiness is a choice," Mel said, echoing David's words from earlier in the day.

"Then go out on your date and make us both happy," Jenny wiped a tear away and smiled bravely.

***

Mel waited outside of the Bella Cucina restaurant, nervously looking to her left, and to her right, hoping to catch a glimpse of Rodney. She wasn't sure what to expect. Certainly not a debonair gentleman in a tuxedo, walking toward her with a rose in hand.

He'll probably be dressed in a clown suit, Mel told herself. *He'll have one of those bicycle horns and he'll start honking it at me. He's going to be a freak. I just know it. Thanks, Jenny. Way to go.*

Then Mel sighed deeply, and resisted the temptation to slap herself.

What's wrong with me? I've already made him out to be a weirdo, and I haven't even met the guy.

She glanced to the left again, and then to the right. No sign of Rodney.

Looking down at her watch, she saw that he was three minutes late already.

Then the door of the restaurant opened.

"Imelda?"

She whirled around at the sound of her name, and there he was.

Rodney.

Just like in the picture Jenny showed her, he was handsome, with spiky blonde hair and deep blue eyes, and a smile that would light up any room. He looked well-groomed and handsome in his chambray shirt and khakis.

Suddenly Mel wasn't so upset to be on a blind date.

"Hi," she said.

"I got here about twenty minutes ago," he said. "So I went inside and got our name on the wait list. They've got our table ready. Come on, I'll show you where it is." He smiled.

Mel smiled and entered the restaurant, taking Rodney's lead.

He even held the door for her.

Not bad, Mel mused. *Polite, kind and thoughtful. What a nice change of pace from that jerk, Devin Ryan.*

Then she smiled. *Maybe this wasn't such a bad idea after all.*

Chapter 10
Wednesday

When Donna woke, she glanced at the clock on her nightstand. It was a little after five in the morning. Her alarm wasn't set to go off until six. A nagging feeling told her something was wrong.

"Yeah," she heard Darius say, in a muffled, hushed voice from the bedroom next to hers. "I wasn't expecting to get out so soon, either."

She sat up, sliding her feet into her bedroom slippers, and tiptoed to the wall. Pressing her ear against it, she struggled to make out her son's words.

"I know, man. It's been a long time. We got a lot of catching up to do."

Darius was obviously talking on the phone. *But who was he talking to? And why in the wee hours of the morning, before the sun had come up?*

"Yeah. Well things have changed. Quite a bit. Got a lot to talk to you about." Darius laughed. "I've missed you too, man."

Donna cringed. Apparently he was talking to one of his old friends.

Oh please, Lord, Donna prayed. *Please don't let it be one of those so-called friends that led him down the wrong path. But then again... what other kind of friends did he have?* She shuddered.

Darius laughed again. "Yeah. Well I can't wait to see you and

Fang. I've missed that dawg!"

Fang? Donna wondered. *What kind of name is that? Probably some street thug he was running with before his days behind bars. And when did it become okay to call your friends 'dawgs?'*

"Alright. Tonight at eight. Just pick me up at the convenience store down the corner from my house."

I think you mean MY house! Donna wanted to storm into his room and cry out. *This is MY home, and you're only living here out of the goodness of my heart! And if you dare start running with the same crowd of criminals and go back to a life of drugs and violence, and you dare bring it into MY home and put your own mother and sister in danger, I'll be throwing you out of my house and that will be it! Don't make me do this, Darius!*

"Okay. Catch you later, man. Peace."

Yeah, I got your peace right here, son, Donna thought to herself, balling up a fist and punching the air. *I brought you into this world and I can take you out!*

Donna heard the soft "beep" as Darius pressed the button to end the phone call. She leaned against the wall and sighed as she recalled their conversation in the car on the way home from the prison, only days ago.

"I'm a changed man, Mama," he had insisted.

"So tell me, how is it that you're different now?" she had asked him.

"I found the Lord while I was in prison."

Donna felt offended. "What are you talking about, son? You've known the Lord all your life. You were raised in a Christian home, with a Christian mother and father. Don't you remember? The bedtime stories we read to you were from the Bible. And as soon as you could walk, we had you down on your knees in prayer. We had you in Sunday School and church every week. And don't you remember – I forced you to keep on going, every Sunday, right up until you moved out. So don't you sit here and tell me that you didn't meet the Lord until you went to prison, Darius." Her tone grew angrier as she spoke.

"I know, Mama. Don't get upset." Darius used the most soothing tone he could. "You did all the right things. And so did Dad, God rest his soul. You both gave me a great spiritual foundation."

"But you mean to tell me that you didn't know the Lord until you were behind bars."

Darius nodded. "God was always waiting just outside my heart, Mama. I just wasn't ready to let him in. Not until I went to prison."

Donna drove in silence for a while. "If that's true, then I'm happy for you," she finally said. "I just can't figure out where I went wrong."

"You didn't. You were always a good, loving, Christian mother. You were a wonderful role model and you taught me all of the right things. It was me who failed, Mama. And it's when I was stripped of everything – my clothes, my money, my friends, my family– that's when I realized that underneath it all, I was just a weak, scared, and lonely person. And that's when I took a good hard look at myself and realized that I needed salvation."

Donna glanced at him out of the corner of her eye. "Is that what you told the parole board? Were those the magic words that got you out early?"

Darius sunk into his seat and sighed. "I know I don't deserve your forgiveness," he said softly. "But if God was willing to forgive me, hopefully you can too, Mama?"

She sighed deeply. "Actions speak louder than words," she said. "If you've changed, don't tell me. Show me."

Tiptoeing back to bed, Donna wondered how secretive phone calls in the early hours of the morning, including the mention of some kind of accomplice named "Fang," could be a sign that Darius had changed his ways.

Shortly after she closed her eyes, her alarm buzzed loudly. Med-Surg South was waiting for its fearless leader to come and take the reins in a little less than two hours. The traffic, glaring news cameras, and reporters that seemed to have overtaken the hospital and every road leading to it had finally died down a bit, but Donna still felt it was best to leave early and allow plenty of travel time as long as Devin Ryan was on her floor. She suspected that any change in his condition, whether good or bad, would trigger another mad rush of media and gawkers to Dogwood Regional. Donna was tired, and for a moment, thought about taking some time off. But then she began to worry about how a typical day would unfold without her being onsite to lead the way. Brad had been in a funk since Sue rejected him. Miriam was obsessed with her new grandson, and her attention was everywhere else but work. Haylie's obsession was Devin Ryan, and Donna had pulled her out of his room more than once to put her back to the task of caring for her own patients. And Mel, poor Mel... heaven only knew what kind of stress and pressure she was under with a pregnant daughter at home and a high-profile celebrity in her care. *Poor Mel.*

They all need a vacation, Donna thought to herself. Then she heard Darius step out of his room, and very quietly, creep down the hallway to leave the house.

And so do I.

***

"So how was your blind date last night?" Jenny asked. "I was too tired to wait up for you and get the report last night," She cupped her hand over her mouth to cover a yawn.

"You went out on a date?" Fourteen-year old Michael asked from across the kitchen as he poured a bowl of cereal and joined his sister and mother at the table in the dining room.

Mel shrugged. "It was okay, I guess."

"Tell me about him," Jenny said excitedly. "Did he look like his picture?"

"Yeah, more or less. He's a handsome guy."

"So tell me about him."

"Well," Mel said, "his name is Rodney. He was born and raised in Dogwood. Did a four year tour of duty in the Army, traveled all over the globe, and came back home after he was done. Now he's working on his MBA during the day, and managing a restaurant at night."

"What restaurant?" Jenny asked.

Mel cringed. "Carolina Fried Chicken and Barbeque."

"Oh, my favorite!" Michael said excitedly. "Dad takes me there on weekends sometimes and we eat Brunswick Stew and hush puppies."

Mel closed her eyes and shook her head.

Jenny couldn't help but laugh. "So does the chicken man know you're a vegetarian?"

"Yes. Trust me, we had that whole conversation when the server brought the menus. He suggested veal, and I went into a rampage."

Jenny doubled over in laughter. "Well, in spite of that, did you have a good time?"

Mel nodded. "I suppose," she said. "He's a smart guy, very kind and polite, and he put up with my vegetarian rant without even breaking a sweat. He's a nice person. He even gave me a ride back home when my car wouldn't start."

"Oh no!" Jenny cried out. "What happened with the car?"

"No clue. When I went to leave, I put the key in the ignition, turned it and nothing happened. Thought it may have been the battery, and Rodney had cables in his car, so he gave me a jump. That didn't work, though. I had to call a towing company to haul it away to a repair shop. So while we were waiting for a tow truck, we went back into the restaurant and had some dessert. Then he drove me home."

"How romantic," Jenny crooned. "A knight in shining armor coming to your rescue. Sir Chicken Man. That's the stuff dreams are made of, Mom."

Michael munched on his cereal and rolled his eyes. "Gross. Don't talk about romance. I'm trying to eat breakfast."

"Oh hush, Mikey. You're going to be late for the bus if you don't slurp down your cereal and get moving," Jenny said to her little brother, trying on a motherly voice for size. Michael took the cue, quickly finishing his breakfast and grabbing his bookbag before he disappeared out the door.

"So where were we?" Jenny asked. "Oh yes... the knight in shining armor part. Tell me more."

Glaring at her, Mel shook her head. "I'm not a big fan of men right now," she said. "Just because I had one nice blind date doesn't mean that I'm ready to forgive and forget everything that your father did to me."

"Rodney isn't Dad," Jenny said sharply. "You can't judge every man by what Dad did."

"I know, Jennifer. But I'm still not excited about jumping into another relationship and risking getting my heart broken again."

"You don't have to jump into a relationship. Just get to know the guy. And have fun in the meantime. That's not too much to ask, is it?"

Mel shrugged. "I don't know. I'm just not sure what I really want. Rodney's a nice guy, and I'll give you kudos for fixing me up with him. I actually did enjoy his company and had a really good time on our date. But...."

"But what, Mom?"

Mel sighed deeply and looked into Jenny's eyes. "There may just be some truth to what you said the other night. You accused me of not being ready to move on. Maybe you were right."

And maybe I'm crazy for actually considering Bruce's request to forgive him, Mel thought to herself.

Frowning, Jenny touched her mother's shoulder. "I'm sorry, Mom," was all that she could say. She leaned forward and hugged her.

"Oh well," Mel whispered, her face pressed to her daughter's. "I probably should go out with Rodney again, and soon. For our own safety."

"Why?"

"Need to make sure he's not an axe murderer," Mel joked. "After all, he knows where I live now."

***

Mel was in a good mood. Maybe it was the wonderful evening she had with Rodney yesterday. Maybe it was from a good night's sleep. Whatever the reason, she didn't mind, and she welcomed the feeling of being refreshed and happy for a change. She decided to be gracious with Devin Ryan today.

"Good morning, Devin," Mel said with a smile as she walked into his room, wondering if he'd catch the transition. This would be the first morning that she hadn't called him Mr. Ryan.

She stopped short when she realized that he wasn't alone in his room. A tall, lanky woman was sitting on the foot of his bed. Mel's eyes first fixed on her high-dollar stiletto heels and followed her bony legs all the way up to an extremely short skirt, wrapped beneath a pricey leather jacket. It was zipped midway up the woman's torso, and where the zipper ended, her chest began. A strategically placed fat diamond dangled from a pendant, drawing the eye in to her cleavage. After the pronounced ridge of collarbone, Mel followed her slender neck up to her face, half of which was obscured behind a curtain of bleach-blonde bob cut. The woman tilted her head toward her shoulder, and gravity drew the long lock of hair away from her face. Mel immediately recognized her.

Venus Palowski was a barely twenty-something A-list actress with dozens of films and television shows to her credit. The entertainment world had embraced her for her bright-eyed, round-faced, all-American girl appearance, which had been replaced almost overnight with her new vampy vixen look and the questionable loss of somewhere between twenty and thirty pounds. Yet, in spite of the total abandonment of her wholesome girl-next-door image, the world only seemed to love her more, and rewarded her with more media attention than any celebrity could ever hope for.

Coming up next... is Venus Palowski expecting a baby, or has she simply gained back the three pounds she lost last week? Mel resisted the urge to gag herself as the memories of cheesy television intros flooded her mind.

"Hello," she said, putting on her best face and greeting Devin's guest with as much courtesy as she could muster.

Venus looked Mel over from head to toe and turned her face toward Devin, pulling the drape of blonde hair over half of her face again. "Is this the one you were telling me about, pookie? Is this the snarky little nurse who's been so mean to you?"

Mel felt as if she'd been kicked in the seat of her pants.

Devin's eyes grew wide. He looked at Mel apologetically. "That's not what I said," he pleaded. "I mean, that's not how I said it."

Venus looked at Mel. "Poor Devin," she said. "First, he gets all banged up in a horrible accident, then he gets hospitalized in this wretched little podunk town in South Carolina—"

"North Carolina," Mel corrected her.

"Oh, what's the difference," Venus snarled, waving her hand in the air as if she were trying to rid the room of a bad odor. "I was just saying, that after all he's suffered through, it seems like he could at least get a nurse who would treat him with some compassion."

"Venus!" Devin yelled at her. "Show some class for a change! She's standing right in front of us! Don't talk about her like she's not here!"

Mel felt her cheeks flush.

Devin looked at her. "Don't listen to any of this, Mel. I did say some things, but she's not telling you the whole story."

Words were on the tip of her tongue. Mel had plenty to say, but kept her mouth shut, knowing that she'd break into tears if she tried to speak.

"Don't pander to her, Devin," Venus said. "I know you and her are friendly now, but really, honey... she's a nobody. Once you get well and get out of here, you can forget all about her and this dreadful place, and rejoin your real friends."

"Venus," he hissed. "That's enough. You have some nerve to call her a nobody. Do I need to remind you that your mother was a truck stop restaurant waitress and your father is serving life in prison? And that you were born in a camper in some small town in Oklahoma? And that your real name is Bertha Jo Buckner?"

The starlet gasped. "I don't know what you're talking about," she said, defensively.

"Well you better figure it out, fast. There are tons of reporters lurking around the hospital and you just never know what might slip out while I'm sedated or in terrible pain... you know, just not in my right mind." Devin narrowed his eyes.

The actress gave Mel a dirty look and stood up. "He's making that up," she said, directing her attention to Mel again. "And if you repeat a word of it to anyone, I'll sue you so fast your head will spin." Then she reached into her handbag and pulled out a cigarette, planting it between her bright red lips.

"This is a non-smoking facility," Mel quickly said.

"I know," the starlet growled. She looked at Devin again. "Before you decide to gossip about me, Devin, just remember, I've got some secrets about you that I'm sure you wouldn't want broadcast around here."

"I wouldn't dream of spreading gossip about you, Venus," Devin said coldly. "I trust we'll both keep our confidences."

With a quick snap of her neck and flip of her hair, the blonde collected her designer handbag and marched out of the room.

"Nice to meet you, Bertha Jo," Mel said under her breath as the actress brushed past her.

Devin looked at her and laughed. "She's a piece of work, isn't she?"

Mel didn't respond. She approached his bedside and pressed the button to inflate his blood pressure cuff, then focused absentmindedly on the cardiac monitor while she waited for the reading.

"Mel?" He said softly. "I'm sorry. I really am. I didn't mean for it to come across like I was saying bad things about you behind your back. I told her that you and I got off to a rocky start, but that we smoothed things over."

"Don't talk to me, Devin," she said coolly. "Don't talk to me unless it's about your health."

"Come on, Mel," he begged. "We had such a great talk yesterday; I felt like we were finally getting to know each other. Don't you see that Venus was just trying to stir things up and make you angry?"

"Why would she even care to make me angry?"

"Because she's jealous."

"Jealous of me? I don't think so. You just heard her say the words yourself. I'm a nobody."

"You are not a nobody," he insisted. "She's jealous of you because I told her I really like you. "

"I'm done with this conversation, Devin. Just drop it, okay?" A beep sounded, and Devin's blood pressure cuff deflated with a noisy *psssshhhhhht* sound.

"I like you," Devin said.

"Your blood pressure is good," Mel said curtly.

"Mel, please."

She went to the foot of his bed and checked for a pulse in the foot of his injured leg. "Wiggle your toes," she commanded. Devin did as he was told.

Then she peeled back his sheet and checked his chest tube.

"Don't be mad. Please."

Mel zeroed in on one of the incisions on his chest, which appeared a bit more inflamed than it had been the day before. She pressed it lightly with her fingertips, feeling the angry warmth of a slight infection creeping into the skin.

"It looks like one of your incisions might be infected. I'll call the doctor and see if he wants to up your dose of antibiotics. Does your chest hurt?"

"Yes, but not there. Here." He pointed to his heart.

"On a scale of one to ten," she began, "with one being no pain and ten being the worst pain imaginable, what number would you rate your pain right now?"

"Ten. But pain medication's not going to touch it."

"Why don't you think pain medicine will help?"

"It's just a broken heart, Mel. The only way I'll feel better is if you're not mad at me."

"Don't play games with me, Devin."

"I'm sorry, Mel. I didn't mean to upset you."

"Fine," she snapped. "You're forgiven. Now please just drop it."

He watched her face. "You're still mad at me."

Throwing her hands up, she laughed. "For crying out loud, Devin, what does it matter? I'm just your nurse. That's all. You'll get well, and you'll go home, back to your real friends, like snotty little Venus Palowski, or... Bertha Jo Butt... whatever her name is... and you'll never see me again."

"Mel! It's Venus who said all of those hateful things, not me! I want to be your friend. And I'd really like to see you again, after I get out of here."

"Devin, please," Mel begged. "We're not going to be friends. That's just not possible. I'm your nurse, and I'm here to do my job, and that's it. I know you're probably not used to getting "no" for an answer from women, but this time you're just going to have to accept it."

He didn't say anything, but his eyes were still pleading.

"I'm going to call your doctor about those antibiotics," Mel said, and left his room, almost running.

***

"Amena? Are you awake?" Brad tapped her shoulder.

She opened her eyes, looked at him, blinked a few times, and closed them."

"How are you feeling? Sleepy, still?"

She nodded.

"Get some rest, then. I'm just here to take vitals and give you your medication this morning."

Her pulse and blood pressure were both a bit lower than they had been the day before, but still within normal limits.

Brad spied the sputum basin next to her pillow and shuddered at the sight of blood in her mucus. More than he'd seen yesterday. When he'd called Amena's doctor, he had ordered a bronchoscopy and CT scan of her lungs. He imagined that she was still pretty tired from all of the procedures the day before.

After reviewing the results, the word was still the same – pneumonia. No cancer, no apparent secondary infections of any kind. Her doctor had assured Brad that the blood was probably coming from her sinuses, which were no doubt irritated and raw from all of the coughing and sneezing.

Still, Brad's inner voice told him that something was wrong.

"Amena?" He asked. "Ms. Benson?" She continued to snooze. She wasn't just drowsy. At this point, she was non-responsive.

"I'm just a little bit concerned about you, my friend," he said. "I'm going to call your doctor again." *And beg for you to be admitted to the ICU*, Brad thought to himself.

In the doorway, he prayed out, and went back to the nurse's station to call Amena's doctor.

***

"Jenny?" Imelda called out when she entered the apartment. The lights were off, and the house was quiet. She could feel that something was wrong.

"In here," Jenny responded from the darkness ahead of her.

Mel stepped, turned on the light switch in the hallway and peered into the tiny living room. Jenny was laying on her back on the sofa with her knees drawn to her chest. Her eyes were puffy and red.

"I tried to call you," Jenny murmured. "I kept getting your voice mail."

"I had my phone turned off. Your father keeps trying to call me and I don't want to deal with him right now. What's wrong?"

"Mom," Jenny said softy, as she began to cry, "I think I'm losing the baby."

Switching into nurse mode, Mel rushed to her daughter's side. She put one hand on Jenny's forehead, the other to her wrist to feel her pulse. "Why? What's happening?"

"I've been having cramps, and when I went to the bathroom, there was blood."

"A lot or a little?" Mel asked.

"I don't know, Mom. What's a lot or a little? I don't remember how much. I just know I saw blood. And I'm scared."

"Come on," Mel said, grasping Jenny's arms and pulling her to a seated position. She found Jenny's bedroom slippers on the floor and slid her feet into them. "Get up," she said. "Let me help you. Be careful, honey. We're going to the hospital."

***

Lingering in the door of Devin's room, Mel asked herself the same question over and over again.

What am I doing here?

Jenny had just been admitted to the Emergency Department, and was waiting to be seen by a provider. Mel knew that she should have stayed with her, but she knew that if she spent another moment thinking about her daughter losing the baby, she would break down and cry.

She couldn't do that in front of Jenny. She had to be strong for her.

She told Jenny that she needed a cup of coffee, and excused herself for a long walk. Long enough for Mel to take a few deep breaths, clear her mind and regain her strength. And she had every intention of taking that long walk, and returning with a cup of coffee in hand.

Only she didn't go to the cafeteria. She walked to Med-Surg South.

What am I doing here? She asked herself again.

The lights were out, but the television was on, casting a soft, flickering glow through the room. Mel advanced a few steps and could see that Devin's face was turned toward the window and his eyes were closed. She watched his chest rise and fall.

He murmured softly in his sleep and clucked his tongue against the roof of his mouth. Then he rolled his head so that he was facing Mel. His eyes were still closed.

I almost like you this way, Mel thought.

She took a few more steps toward him, until she was standing next to his bed. She found herself leaning toward him.

This was the closest that she'd been to him yet.

She noticed for the first time that there were lines etched into his forehead and around his eyes. Faint though they were, the telltale signs of middle age were still there. She also noticed a crescent-shaped scar just above his eyebrow. His lips were parted, and Mel noticed that one of his bottom teeth was slightly chipped. He had a tiny pink mole under his left nostril, barely visible through the layer of scruffy beard and moustache that was growing on his face.

Wow.

She'd never realized that a person's imperfections could be so endearing. For the first time, she could see Devin Ryan.

Not Devin Ryan, the obnoxious, self-worshipping celebrity, but

Devin Ryan, the imperfect, vulnerable human being, with all of his dings, dents and scratches.

And in the blink of an eye, her feelings about Devin Ryan had changed.

She didn't exactly like him. It wasn't that.

But she wanted to like him.

What's wrong with me? She wondered. *Have I lost my mind? He's my patient! And he's a jerk to boot! So what am I doing gawking at him while he sleeps? My daughter may be losing her baby right now, and I'm here, with Devin Ryan? Have I lost my mind? What is WRONG WITH ME?*

Repulsed at herself, she turned to leave.

"Mel?"

No! You're not supposed to be awake! She whirled back around. "I thought you were asleep," she said.

Devin shook his head. "Nah. Just resting, that's all."

Embarrassed, Mel took a step closer to the door. "I'm sorry, Devin. You need to get your rest. I'll go."

"Please don't," he begged, propping himself up on his elbows.

For some reason she couldn't put her finger on, she relented, and turned on the lights as she walked back into his room. She sank down into the chair next to his bed. "I'm really sorry. I thought I was being quiet when I came in."

"You were," he said. "I couldn't hear you at all."

"So how did you know I was here?"

"I smelled you. The fragrance you wear, whatever it is. It smells like plumeria."

She felt herself blushing. "It's just lotion." she said. "Wearing latex gloves and washing your hands all day dries them out, so I keep a bottle of lotion in my locker." She held one of her hands up to her face and sniffed it. Indeed, it did smell – very faintly – of plumeria.

"Those are the traditional flowers that they use for leis in Hawaii," Devin said. "I lived there for eight months. My last movie was filmed in Honolulu."

"I think I saw the previews for that one," Mel said. "Honolulu Hitman, right?"

"In spite of the ridiculous movie title, it really wasn't one of the stupid ones," he said with a chuckle.

They sat in silence for a moment.

"I'm sorry," they both said at the same time.

They laughed.

"Let me go first," Mel said. "I've been incredibly rude to you, and I apologize. I'm a really angry and upset person right now, Devin, and while it has nothing to do with you, I've been taking it out on you. I'm appalled with myself. I've been very unprofessional with some of the things that I've said, and the way that I've acted. I'm ashamed."

"It's okay," he insisted. "Apology accepted, but totally unnecessary. I haven't really acted appropriately toward you either, Mel. I feel horrible. I've been hitting on you since I met you. I keep telling myself that it's not the time and place, but every time you walk into the room, I forget all that, and I just kind of lose my head. I know you probably think I'm an idiot, but I just can't help it. You're beautiful, and smart, and honest, and every time you're near me, my heart starts pounding."

"Yeah, I noticed that. You're hooked up to a cardiac monitor." She felt herself blushing.

He laughed softly, and then there was awkward silence.

"How about this," Devin suggested, "Can we just start all over again? Just pretend we haven't yet met? And that way we'll have a fresh start. Today can be our new beginning."

Mel pondered his proposal. "Okay," she said.

He stretched out his hand to her. "Hi, I'm Devin Ryan."

She shook hands with him. "Imelda Tagaro," she said. "My friends call me Mel."

"Pleased to meet you, Mel."

Don't smile, don't smile, don't smile, she commanded herself. But she couldn't help it.

"Now that we're off to a fresh start," he said, "it looks like you've got a lot on your mind right now. Anything you want to talk about?"

No thanks, was what Mel wanted to say. But when she opened her mouth, different words came out, followed by a rush of tears. "Everything in my life is just so screwed up right now," she wept.

Devin looked at her sympathetically. "Well let's talk about it. Tell me what's wrong."

"Everything," Mel cried.

"So then pick a starting place, and you can cover it all."

"Okay," Mel said, "My daughter, Jenny, just dropped out of college and moved back home because she's pregnant. The father of her child has disappeared off the face of the earth, and I don't know how in the world I'm going to come up with the money to pay for her medical bills. I asked my idiot ex-husband, Bruce, for help, but it turns out that he's broke because the woman he left me for a couple of years ago maxed out his credit cards. My best friend, Brad, is completely depressed because his fiancée just left him, and he's totally withdrawn. We haven't said two words to each other in a week, and I'm worried about him, but I don't know what to do to help, because he's totally shut me out." Tears were pouring down her cheeks.

"Oh Mel," Devin said softly.

"And the whole reason that I'm here right now? I just brought Jenny to the Emergency Department a few minutes ago, and she may be losing her baby."

"Mel," he said softly. "I'm so sorry."

"I'm mad," she said. "And sad, and worried, and scared, and lonely, and I don't want to feel this way anymore. And I shouldn't be venting like this to you. You're a patient; I'm your nurse... it's unprofessional."

"Mel, stop," he said firmly. "Stop beating yourself up. You keep calling yourself a nurse like it means you're supposed to be some kind of god. You're still human. And so am I. We both have feelings and fears and things we have to deal with. Just because you're my nurse and I'm your patient doesn't mean that we can't relate to each other as people. Take away the roles and the titles, and we're just friends." He paused. "That is, if you want us to be. And in case you haven't noticed, I could really use a friend right now. It gets lonely when you're stuck in a hospital bed."

She looked at him, almost amused. "But you've got all of these people breezing in and out of your room all day. Your publicist, the occasional fan who sneaks past security and all the other hospital staff who linger around and chat with you... and don't forget your dear friend Venus..."

Devin shook his head. "They're not friends," he corrected her. "They're just here to gawk. Or to have something to brag about to their friends, or to the press. I've had so many cameras flash in my face, and I've signed so many autographs, I feel like I'm trapped in celebrity hell. It's like being on display at an unpaid gig... actually, a gig that I am going to have to pay for!"

Mel frowned. "I guess being in the spotlight all the time isn't easy."

"You can say that again," Devin groaned. "But I hope you don't think I'm trying to trivialize your problems. I certainly didn't mean to make this conversation about me."

"No, of course not," Mel said. Then she smiled. "It's actually kind of nice to put my problems out of my mind for a minute. So let's keep talking about you."

Devin sighed. "I wouldn't know where to begin. What do you want me to talk about?"

Mel thought for a moment. "Who's the real Devin Ryan?" She asked. "When you take off the movie star mask, who are you really? Where do you come from? What's your family like? What makes you happy... and sad?"

He grinned. "Tough questions. I knew you wouldn't go easy on me. Okay, for starters, family. I was born and raised in Florida. My father died before I was born, so I was raised by my mom, Beverly. She never remarried so I never had a Dad, or any brothers or sisters. My father's parents were from Massachusetts. I only met them a few times as a kid and don't remember them very much. Dad was an only child, so I'm the last Ryan. On my mom's side, her father passed away when I was young, and I don't remember him. Mom's mother has Alzheimer's and is in a nursing home. My mom has a brother and a sister, and I've got four cousins, but since we're spread out all over the country , I don't get to see them often."

"So you've got a really small family."

"Mom and I… that's pretty much it."

"You never married or had children?"

"No."

"Don't mean to pry, but why not?"

"Never found the right woman. My mom has been the only lady in my life for as long as I can remember. She's the only woman that I've ever been close to. Or really loved, for that matter. Hopefully you'll get to meet her. She's flying up here tomorrow to come and visit."

"I never would have pegged you for a Mama's Boy," Mel teased. "But seriously, I'd love to meet her."

"So back to my interrogation," Devin joked, "You asked what makes me happy… and sad. The happy part is easy. A lot of things make me happy. Simple things. Like a good deep dish pizza. Riding in a convertible on a sunny day with the top down. A day at the beach, when it's hot enough to fry eggs on the sidewalk. And kids. I love kids. I enjoy being around kids more than I do adults these days."

Mel thought back to seeing images of Devin on the TV and in tabloids with children at charity events. "You volunteer with one of those foundations that grants wishes to sick children who want to meet their favorite actors, don't you?"

Devin's face lit up. "It's called the 'Wish Upon a Movie Star' foundation. I did in the past, yes. I've been so busy filming movies lately that I haven't had as much time to devote to the kids as I'd like. But that's going to change once I get out of here."

Mel felt ashamed for looking at Devin as a drunken, chain-smoking playboy. She wondered why it had been so easy to forget about the photos of him at the bedsides of sick children, sharing his time and boosting their spirits. "That's really wonderful, Devin."

"I'd love to have a kid of my own someday." He pointed toward the wall behind Mel. "See the card taped next to the window? Take it down and hand it to me, if you don't mind." Mel reached behind her and retrieved the card. On the front of it was a duck in a wheelchair. The pictures and the message inside the card had been scrawled by a very young hand, almost illegibly so, but Devin had no problem reading it.

"Dear Devin Ryan," He began, "Please get well soon so you can finish making your movie. I am proud you are making a movie in my town because you are my hero. I make a wish for you every morning when I wake up and I say a bedtime prayer for you every night. So get well okay? You mean the whole world to me. Your number one fan, Justin Creech." When Devin finished reading, he closed the card and held it in his hands for a moment, treasuring the words of the young fan.

"How sweet," Mel said.

He nodded. "I've received a ton of fan mail since I've been here. So much that they're running out of space in the mailroom to hold all of the cards and letters and gifts that fans have been sending. I've been opening and reading as many of them as I can, and the hospital volunteers are moving them out of my room just as quickly as they're coming in, because they could probably fill this room if they didn't. But this one card just meant so much to me, Mel. I had to keep it in here, where I could see it."

Slowly but surely, Mel was opening her eyes to the real Devin.

"You asked me what makes me sad," Devin said. "My past. I've done a lot of stupid and crazy things. I was teetering on the edge, Mel. All those pictures and videos you've seen of me... that's who I used to be. I was a chauvinist pig who used women, and I was a rude, callous jerk to everyone that I came into contact with. And I was addicted to alcohol and strung out on cocaine. I was so miserable that I tried to kill myself with an overdose. It was Venus who found me, passed out on my sofa with a suicide note in my pocket. That's my big 'secret' that she alluded to today. I was hospitalized, and a few days later, sent to a substance abuse treatment program. It helped me get my life back together. It was all kept out of the media, so very few people really know about that part of me, that I hit rock bottom. And very few people know that for nearly a year now, I've been clean and sober."

Mel sat quietly, holding back tears.

"I went to hell and came back, Mel, and I never want to go there again. Those days are over for me. I'm ashamed of the person I used to be. I hurt a lot of people, my mother the most. I never thought she'd forgive me, but she did, and we're closer now than we've ever been. It's amazing how loving and strong mothers can be for their children."

Reaching for the tissue dispenser on the wall, Mel knew that it was pointless trying to fight off tears.

Devin looked at the card again. "And it's amazing that people really thought I was some big star and role model, when really, I was just a giant screw-up. When I read Justin Creech's note, I realized what a tremendous responsibility I have to him, and every other child out there who thinks I'm a hero. I owe it to him to be a better man. So I asked one of the volunteers to put Justin's card on the wall, to remind me that my goal every single day is to wake up and try to be a man worthy of receiving it."

Burying her face in a pile of tissue, Mel wept.

"Oh... hey...I didn't mean to make you cry," Devin said.

Blotting the corners of her eyes, Mel shook her head. "Don't feel bad," she said. "It's not your fault."

Devin watched her, his face filled with worry. "I'm sorry. I know your daughter is in the Emergency Department. I hope I'm not upsetting you and making things worse."

"You're not at all," Mel said. "And I know I need to be with her, but Devin, I'm so scared it's going to be bad news. I don't know what I'll do if it is."

"It'll be okay, Mel," he said. "Whatever happens, you and your family will get through it."

She covered her face with a fresh tissue, hoping to wipe off all traces of her breakdown. "The irony in this is unreal," she said. "When Jenny first told me she was pregnant, I was devastated. I was hoping it was some sort of joke, or maybe just a bad dream. And when I found out it wasn't, I was still hoping that she was wrong. Right up until she went to the doctor's office, I was hoping that they'd do an ultrasound and say that there was no baby, and they'd tell her that it was just a big mistake; that the pregnancy tests had been false negatives and all of the pregnancy symptoms must have been caused by stress."

Devin frowned.

"But that wasn't the case. When I saw the ultrasound picture, I knew the baby was real, and whether it was planned or not didn't matter. Jenny was going to be a mother, and I was going to be a grandmother. She had a tiny little life inside of her, and it was going to be part of our family. And now that she's lying in an Emergency bed, waiting to be seen for a possible miscarriage, the only thing in the world that matters to me is keeping the baby alive." Mel stopped and laughed. "Isn't that ridiculous? Just a few days ago, I was trying my best to wish the baby out of existence. Now I'd give anything just to be certain it's going to live."

Devin smiled. "Not at all. I can't imagine feeling any other way."

"I feel like I've lost my mind. I don't know what I'm supposed to think – or feel – about anything anymore."

"Hey," Devin said softly, and reached out his hand toward her. She stared at him for a moment, and then gave hers in return. He squeezed it. "I'm so sorry, Mel," he said. "Whatever happens, I hope you know that I care and I'm here if you need a friend." He pointed to his leg in traction. "I'm not going anywhere."

"Yes, I think it's safe to say you're stuck here for a while."

"Can I tell you something that I've noticed about you, Mel?"

She sat upright. "I guess so."

"You put everyone else first. In the wonderful world of show biz, everyone you meet looks out for themselves, and only themselves. I've never met anyone like you. You just opened up and shared your worries with me, and they weren't about you. They were all about your family and your friends. I can't imagine how such a big heart could fit into such a tiny person, but I just want you to know I admire you." He squeezed her hand.

She looked away. "I need to get back to Jenny," she said, gently pulling her hand from his. "Thank you for the talk. I'm really glad I came up here, Devin."

"So… why did you come up here?"

"Just… you know… I was just checking up on my patient."

"You're off the clock, though." A grin slowly spread across his face.

"Bye Devin," she said, as she tried not to smile. She shut off the lights as she left his room.

***

Back at the Emergency Department, Mel cautiously approached the door to Jenny's room, and sent up a prayer of hope before she entered.

Please let my grandchild be alive and well. Take anything else away from me if need be, but please don't take this baby away.

She knocked. "Come in," Jenny's voice beckoned from behind the door.

Mel entered to find Jenny in a blue checkered hospital gown, sitting on the side of the bed, her legs dangling toward the floor.

Behind her, a young woman in a white coat listened to Jenny's lungs with a stethoscope. Mel had seen her around the hospital a few times. Glancing at her nametag, she learned that her name was Sarah Fullbright, and that she was a nurse practitioner.

"You must be Jenny's mom. Have a seat," she said.

Mel crossed the room and sank into a chair in the corner. She watched as Sarah finished Jenny's exam.

After shucking off her gloves and washing her hands, she turned to Mel and shook hands with her. "I'm Sarah," she said.

"Imelda. Or Mel if you prefer. Nice to meet you."

"You work here, don't you?" Clearly, Sarah had recognized her too.

"Yes. I'm a nurse on Med-Surg South."

Sarah nodded. "It's good to meet you, Mel." Then she turned her attention to Jenny. "Is it okay if I share with your mom what I just told you?"
Jenny nodded.

"It seems that you brought Jenny here with some bleeding, and that both of you were afraid that she was having a miscarriage, is that right?"
Mel nodded, feeling her heart pound.

Sarah continued. "Well, we did an ultrasound and some lab work. The baby appears to be doing fine."

Mel sighed in relief.

"The major concerns if we see bleeding in the second semester is that there may be a problem with the placenta, or that the cervix may be trying to dilate too early. But I'm not seeing either of those things happening. The bleeding isn't significant, from what I can tell, and it's probably due to a mild inflammation of some kind. I performed a pelvic exam on Jenny and couldn't find anything that worried me. Her labs were all normal, and the ultrasound looked just fine."

Tears of relief began to fall from Mel's eyes. "So the baby's fine?" She asked, making sure she understood.

"Baby's fine," Sarah nodded emphatically. "I've asked Jenny to make an appointment with her OB-GYN in a few days for a follow-up, just to make sure everything still looks good, but from what I can tell, all is well. Mom and baby are going to be alright."

Mel leaped out of the chair and wrapped her arms around Jenny. "Thank God," she said softly, as she buried her face in Jenny's neck.

"Do you have any questions?" Sarah asked.

"I don't," Jenny said.

"The baby's okay. That's all I need to know," Mel said.

Jenny yawned. "Let's go home. I'm beat."

Chapter 11
Thursday

"I thought we could do something fun today," Mel said excitedly. "Let's get out of here for a little while."

Devin's eyes grew wide. "Are you serious? Is that even possible? With my leg in traction and the chest tube and the whole nine yards?"

Mel grinned. "Not exactly," she said. "You're staying put for a while, right where you are. But lucky for you, I'm here to take you on a journey via the wonderful world of imagination."

Devin arched one eyebrow. "Okay, you've got my attention. What does this involve?"

"Close your eyes."

"Uh... okay." Devin smiled.

Mel reached into her pocket and pulled out her MP3 player and a small set of portable speakers, placing them on the rolling tray next to Devin's bed. She skipped through her playlists until she found the one that she'd put together the evening before. She hit the play button and the sound of crashing waves and the occasional cry of seagulls filled the room. She watched Devin's face, and was overjoyed to see him begin to smile.

The gentle sound of an acoustic guitar faded in, as the waves crashing faded out into the background.

Then Mel took out a small bottle of sea salt-scented oil and uncapped it. She placed it on the edge of the rolling tray, and gently moved it closer toward Devin.

"Keep your eyes closed," she said. "But take a deep breath."

Devin's grin grew even wider when he smelled the oil. "Wow," he said.

"So keeping your eyes closed, why don't you tell me where you are?"

"Where *we* are," Devin corrected her. "I'm not going anywhere unless you're coming with me. I'm still in pretty bad shape. I think I need my nurse by my side."

"Okay then," Mel chuckled. "Tell me where we are."

"In Hawaii. On the beach, of course."

Mel took a flashlight out of her bag. It had a piece of bright orange transparent film taped over the bulb. Michael had used it in elementary school for a science project, to simulate how the sun casts light on the earth. Mel placed the flashlight on its end on Devin's table, pointing the light toward the ceiling. She switched it on, and a sunny orange glow filled the room. Mel knew that Devin would be able to sense the change in color, even behind closed eyes.

"And what do you see?"

"The sun's shining It's a beautiful day."

They sat silently for a few moments, and Mel studied his face. His smile never left.

"What else do you see?"

"Blue water. Beautiful, crystal blue water"

"And do you want to go for a swim?"

"I'd absolutely love to."

Mel turned off the flashlight, and pulled one more item out of her bag.

A baby mobile. An early gift for the baby, of course, but she didn't think that Jenny would mind Devin getting some use out of it first. The mobile wasn't the traditional kind that attached to a crib and suspended overhead with tiny objects dangling from strings. It was a tiny, battery-operated projector, which Mel turned on with the flip of a switch. Swirling patterns of blue, green, and silvery waves, with smiling fish and turtles appeared on the ceiling, and began to rotate in a giant circle around the room.

Mel stood and crossed the room to the light switch and turned the lights off. Then she drew the shades closed. The light show on the ceiling was breathtaking.

As she returned to her seat next to Devin's bed, she took in a whiff of salty air from the fragrant oil, and took a moment to admire her creation, as one beach song finished and another began.

"Okay, Devin. We just swam all the way out in the middle of the Pacific. And now we're under water, all the way at the bottom of the ocean. Open your eyes."

Devin's eyes opened, and grew wide when he saw the shimmering waves and swimming fish and turtles above him.

For a moment, he was speechless. He took a few deep breaths.

"Mel," he finally said, "This is amazing. Thank you. Thank you so much."

"You're welcome, Devin."

They sat silently, and Mel watched Devin's heart monitor. His heart rate was slower than it had been when she first walked into the room, but it suddenly began to pick up a bit. An irregular rhythm appeared for a split second, but corrected itself. His breathing seemed deeper, each breath almost a sigh. She watched him closely, wondering if something was wrong.

Then he sniffled.

And reached up to his face, touching his eyes.

Uh oh… is he crying? Mel wondered. A slew of questions were on the tip of her tongue: *Is something wrong? Was the beach idea a bad idea? What's your pain on a scale of one to ten?*

"I want you to know something," he said, seeming to choke on his words. "Sorry, I guess I'm getting emotional here…"

"Yes?"

He paused.

"There's nowhere else I'd rather be right now, than here at the bottom of the ocean with you."

Mel smiled. "I'm glad," she said.

"I want us to go together," Devin said. "When I'm well, and maybe not all the way to the ocean floor," he laughed. "The shore would do just fine."

Mel laughed. "I figured," she said. "You know, I just might enjoy that, Devin."

"Really?"

"Yeah."

"So it's a date," he said. "I can't think of any better motivation to get well. A day on the beach with the girl I love—"

"Whoa," Mel said, and jumped up from her seat.

"I'm sorry," he said, jolting upright. "I didn't mean to say that. I was just…I don't know… I'm sorry, Mel."

Mel stood silently for a moment. "You're on a lot of pain medication," she laughed. "It's not the first time someone mistook a morphine buzz for love."

"I'm not buzzed, Mel. I shouldn't have said that. I was just enjoying myself so much that the filter between my brain and my mouth didn't catch that thought, and I'm so incredibly sorry for killing the moment."

"It's okay," Mel said, snatching up her things and packing them back in her bag. "Maybe this was a bad idea, Devin. I think I've crossed a line. I shouldn't have gotten so close to you. I've given you the wrong idea—"

"No, Mel, it was a great idea. You've done everything right. Everything. I hope you can forgive me. Please."

"It's fine, Devin. You haven't done anything wrong."

"So why are you leaving?"

"I've got other patients. If you need anything, I'll send Haylie in."

"Mel… I'm sorry!" He called out as she rushed out the door.

***

Later that evening, when she got home, Mel sank into the sofa and rested her heels on the coffee table. She took a few deep breaths before turning on the TV. Flipping through the channels, all that she could find was celebrity gossip shows and news, and everyone abuzz about Devin Ryan, and how the filming schedule in Dogwood had been delayed due to his injury. The next channel she found featured a Devin Ryan movie marathon, in tribute to the downed hero.

Mel shook her head and shut off the television. Closing her eyes, she took a hint from Miriam and tried a thirty-second escape, conjuring up the same image of a hunky man named Hans giving her a shoulder massage.

Only in her mind, Hans looked like Devin.

"Oh my God," she groaned. "I'm falling for him."

Her cell phone rang in her pocket and she sighed, wondering when Bruce would take the hint and quit calling. She let the call go to voice mail.

Moments later, it rang again.

Stupid Bruce, she sighed, and let the call go to voice mail once again.

After only a few seconds, the phone rang again.

"That's it," she grumbled. "You're getting a piece of my mind!" She pressed the "talk" button on her phone and held it to her ear. "WHAT?" she screamed.

There was a brief pause on the other end of the line.

"Shoo-wop, shoo-wah," sang four male voices, barber-shop quartet style, "Shoo-wop, shoo-wah,"

"A-weee-oooh," a tenor voice sailed in.

"Shoo-wop, shoo-wah, shoo-wap, shoo-wah-ah…"

Mel couldn't help it. A smile overtook her face. She cupped her hand over her mouth to keep from laughing. One of the male voices departed from the shoo-wopping and sang:

I'm so sorry, sweetheart

Your feelings are hurt

I hope you'll forgive me

For acting like a jerk

Shoo-wop, shoo-wah, shoo-wop, shoo-wah…

A new voice carried the next few lines:

Well I'm just a patient

And you are my nurse

I overstepped my boundaries

And I acted like a jerk, oh…

Shoo-wop, shoo-wah, shoo-wop, shoo-wah…

Mel felt a blush spreading across her cheeks and down her neck like wildfire. After another chorus of shoo-wopping, a deeper male voice jumped in:

I wish I could take back

When I said the "L-word"

Doesn't mean I don't mean it

It just means that I'm a jerk

Shoo-wop, shoo-wah, shoo-wop, shoo-wah…

Mel couldn't stand it any longer. She doubled over in laughter as the *shoo-whops* poured through the earpiece of her cell phone. One last male voice jumped, and she knew it was Devin's:

I hope you'll forgive me

I know I've been crass

But I can't help it, darling,

'Cause you know I'm just a…

Jerk…

Oh, shoo-wop, shoo-wah… shoo-wop, shoo-wah…

"Devin," Mel laughed. "Oh, Devin…"

The crooners finished their song, with a tenor capping off the performance with another high-note "Ooooh-weee-ooooh-ooooh-ooooh."

Mel put down the phone to clap loudly, then picked it back up again. "How did you get my cell number?" She asked.

"I didn't," he swore. "Haylie did the dialing. Mel heard Haylie giggle nervously in the background. "Is she mad?" She asked.

"No, tell her I'm not," Mel said. "Who's there singing with you, anyway?"

"Oh, it's just the Dogwood Regional Medical Center barbershop quartet," he said.

"I didn't know we had one," Mel laughed.

"Well, you didn't – until today. My publicist was bored, so I put him to work scouting talent around the hospital. He pulled together a nice bunch. We've got... let's see... Haylie's beau, Dan... then we've got Bob, a Respiratory Therapist, Charlie from Environmental Services, and me, the resident jerk patient from Med-Surg South."

"And who wrote the incredibly specific lyrics?"

"Well, that would be me," Devin confessed. "Have I earned your forgiveness yet, or should I keep going?"

"Devin," Mel laughed, "you're not a jerk, and you've done nothing that calls for forgiveness, and if you don't stop asking for it, then you'll really be in trouble."

"Hmmmm," he said thoughtfully. "So if I'm hearing you loud and clear, it sounds like I'm overdoing it."

"Maybe just a bit," she said, "but I want you to know, that was the sweetest thing that any man has ever done for me. I've never been serenaded. And no one has ever written a song for me before."

"Do you like it? It's called "I'm a Jerk," and I wrote it on one of those disposable toilet seat liners from the bathroom because we couldn't find anything else to write on. You can keep it, if you like."

Mel laughed so hard she nearly dropped the phone. "Save it for me, please," she said. "I think it deserves a special place in my scrapbook. You're amazing, Devin."

"Promise you're not mad at me?"

"Not at all. And even if I was, you would have completely redeemed yourself by now."

"Fantastic. Well, I don't want to keep you, Mel. Go rest up and spend some time with your kids, and I'll see you tomorrow. And if you get bored, there's a Devin Ryan Stupid Movie Marathon on one of the movie channels tonight. You should check it out. Good stuff."

"I just may," Mel said.

"Good. I'll just be hanging out here. Mom's flying in tonight. You'll get to meet her in the morning."

"I'm looking forward to it. Sleep tight."

"You too. Good night, beautiful girl."

Butterflies took over Mel's belly. And the words "I love you" were on the tip of her tongue. She pressed her lips together until the urge to say them went away.

"Good night, Devin."

Chapter 12
Friday

Mel awoke with a smile on her face.

Throughout the night, she dreamed about Devin. They were on a tropical island, standing on an outdoor dance floor in the middle of a crowd. To one side of them, waves crashed on the beachfront. To the other, a live band played, and twinkling multicolored lights were strung up between palm trees. Devin's strong arms were wrapped around her waist, and his cheek was pressed against hers. She could feel his warm breath on her neck, and the stubble of his beard grazed her face as he smiled, a very wide grin from ear to ear.

She wore a long, beautiful dress from the junior's store in the mall. She couldn't believe that Jenny had talked her into buying it, but she had to admit, it did look great on her. So what if she was forty years old? If she could still wear a size six and look good in it... well, why not?

Devin kept telling her how wonderful she smelled. A plumeria flower was tucked behind her ear.

The live band began to play a tango. Devin pulled Mel flush to his body, locked her into a tango-stance, and together, they crept across the dance floor with long, dramatic steps, sharp turns, slow dips, with an occasional flick of Devin's head from side to side, and a toss of Mel's long black hair over her shoulder.

She felt so young and free again.

Even the terrorists couldn't ruin it when they arrived on the scene. Four burly rebels ran onto the dance floor with machine guns and began to fire rounds at her and Devin. Upon hearing the gunfire, the rest of the crowd had disappeared. Only Mel and Devin remained on the dance floor.

Still dancing the tango, he whipped Mel around in a carefully choreographed manner so that she missed all of the bullets, and he caught them for her on his bullet-proof vest. The terrorists, after running out of ammunition, quickly saw that four-to-one was not a favorable enough ratio against Devin Ryan and they disappeared into the night. Mel sighed with relief.

But it didn't last for long. At least a dozen, if not more, ropes dropped to the dance floor from some unseen location above their heads. Ninjas, clad in black uniforms from head to toe, shimmied down the ropes and rushed at her and Devin with swords, throwing stars, and martial arts moves that were impossible to perform without the aid of hidden cables and stunt doubles.

But with the same style and grace that he had used to defeat the terrorist gunmen, Devin dipped Mel at the waist and extended his leg behind him to counterbalance their weight as a couple. As he spun them around in an extremely sexy dance move, his leg knocked down all of the ninjas in one swoop.

Mel sighed delightedly. Just as the tango neared its end, a spaceship landed on the dancefloor, and a clan of creepy-looking aliens climbed out, zapping at them with fluorescent green rays of light. Devin reached into Mel's hair and swiftly drew out the bobby pin that was holding her plumeria in place, and with a firm snap of the wrist, it magically extended to become a glowing saber of light. As he spun her around once more, he batted the aliens' lethal light beams back with his own, causing the outer space visitors and their spaceship to burst into flames.

As the roasting aliens and their spacecraft burned down in the background, Devin dipped Mel once again, and gave her a dramatic, *Gone With the Wind*-style kiss.

"Mah hero," Mel whispered with a Southern belle accent.

"My beautiful girl," Devin purred back. Mel could still hear his voice as her eyes opened to the morning sunlight shining through her bedroom window.

Mel sprung to her feet and laughed out loud. Then, Jenny burst into her room, hair mussed and a toothbrush dangling from one side of her mouth. "Mom, what's going on? Are you okay?"

"I'm great, honey. GREAT."

Jenny stared at her. "I heard you laughing. What's up with that?"

"I just woke up from the most amazing dream. It was funny. And sweet. Like a really good movie. The kind you want to see over and over again, because it makes you happy. It makes you laugh."

"You? Laugh?" Jenny's eyebrows shot up on her forehead. "You've been in such a foul mood lately that I thought you had a moratorium on laughter."

"Quit picking on me," Mel said playfully.

Jenny took a step back. "Who are you and what have you done with my mother?"

"Oh come on, Jenny."

Jenny's eyes grew wide as she suddenly dropped her toothbrush, cupped her hand over her mouth and gagged while she made a beeline to the bathroom.

"That's what you get for picking on me!" Mel shouted after her. "Don't worry, Jen, the morning sickness should be fading away soon."

***

During the morning drive to work, traffic was heavy and it took Mel ten minutes longer than it usually did to arrive at work. In the parking deck and on the hospital lawn, reporters and news crews were lurking, as were lots of people who didn't seem to be affiliated with the media. Some of them looked like locals.

What's going on? Mel wondered, as she brushed through the crowd of reporters. As they saw her approaching in her scrubs, she plugged a set of earphones into her ears and turned up her mp3 player. She set the playlist to the same set of beachy tunes that she had played for Devin the day before.

Mel smiled as she remembered the words he'd said.

... a day at the beach with the girl I love...

Although her initial response had been somewhat of a panic, her heart melted a little more every time the words echoed through her mind.

I feel like I'm back in junior high school, she thought, as she dodged news crews and made her way through the front door, resisting the urge to skip down the hallway and into the elevator.

She wondered how Devin would respond when she told him that she had feelings for him too. She was a bit too cautious to call it love, but something was definitely there. She would tell him that morning.

And she would tell him that whenever he was ready and all healed up, she would accept his offer and go to the oceanfront with him. Any beach, anywhere in the world.

It's a date, she would say with a wink and a smile.

When the elevator doors opened and she stepped out onto the floor of Med-Surg South, she could feel the tension immediately. Flashing her hospital ID as she pushed past two security guards, she knew that something was wrong.

Donna, Brad, Haylie and Miriam clustered at the nurse's desk, looking very serious as they spoke with the hospital's director of public relations.

Public relations? Mel wondered. *Maybe Venus Palowski came back and pulled some kind of crazy stunt to grab some publicity for herself.*

Donna looked up and met Mel's gaze, and her expression morphed into one of pure anguish.

"Donna? What's going on?" Mel pulled the earphones out of her ears and looked around, confused.

Donna took her by the arm and led her into the break room. "You haven't heard?" She asked.

Mel grew worried. "No. What's going on?"

Donna's eyes grew wide. "Honey... Devin coded last night."

Mel's knees felt wobbly, and for a moment, she felt as if she might faint. "But they brought him back, didn't they? Tell me that they resuscitated him..."

Donna slowly shook her head from side to side. "Mel, I'm sorry..."

"No," Mel said. "That's impossible." She pushed past Donna and into Devin's room. It was empty. Devin's balloons, flowers, and get well cards had been cleared out. The bed was made up for a new patient.

Donna walked into the room behind her and shut the door.

"Oh, I get it," Mel smiled as she spun around. "This is just for the press, right? He's faking his death so they'll leave him alone. Right?"

Donna shook her head again. "Mel," she said softly, "He died just a little after one o'clock this morning. They're going to do an autopsy today, but the doctor thinks he threw a clot and it went to his heart."

Mel shook her head. "That's bull," she said. "I don't believe it."

"Take the day off, Mel," Donna said. "Just go home. Get some rest. Please. I don't think you need to be here today."

"I'm not going anywhere," she replied angrily. "He was fine, Donna. He was fine. Just yesterday, he was laying right here in this bed, alert and conscious, talking and laughing... his spirits were good, he said he wasn't in any pain..."

"That was yesterday," Donna said firmly. "But he's gone now, Mel. And I'm so sorry, I know you got close to him, and I'm so sorry, Honey... but that's the reality we have to face."

"No," Mel shook her head. "No."

"Please," Donna begged. "Go home, Mel." She opened the door and stood next to it.

"I don't understand," Mel said, walking out of Devin's room. At the nurse's station, Brad touched her shoulder. "Mel, I'm sorry," he said.

She shook her head. "Not now," she said. "Just... stop. Don't. I don't want to talk about it right now." Her eyes were brimming with tears.

"There's someone you should meet," Miriam said, motioning toward a petite woman sitting on a visitor's bench in the hallway. Her salt-and-pepper colored hair was covering most of her face from Mel's point of view.

"Beverly?" Miriam called out.

Upon hearing her name, the woman stood and reached up to her face, brushing her long bangs back with her fingers and securing them behind her ear. Mel felt as if, once again, she was looking into Devin's eyes. Miriam could see that no introduction was necessary.

As she approached the nurse's station, Mel's eyes grew wide. "Miriam, what am I supposed to say to her?"

Miriam placed her hands on Mel's shoulders and drew her close. "There are a million wrong things you can say," she explained. "Like 'he's in a better place now' or 'I know how you feel' or 'it's a good thing he's not in pain and suffering anymore.' I know you feel the need to say something meaningful, Mel, but you don't have to. The most important thing that you can do is just be there for her. Your presence is what matters most right now, and she'll let you know what she needs from you. It might be a hug, or a hand to hold, or someone to listen to her tell stories about Devin when he was a child, or just to sit quietly with her for a moment while she cries."

Mel nodded, blinking tears away from her eyes.

"And if you need to say something," Miriam continued, "just tell her how you feel – that you're very sorry for her loss."

Mel stepped forward and whispered into Miriam's ear. "That's his mother, Miriam. Oh my God... can you imagine losing a child?"

"No," Miriam said, beginning to choke up. "I can't imagine. Go be with her, Mel. She needs you. You've been taking care of Devin all this time, and the way that you continue to care for him is that you're there for his family. Now your job is to be a healer to his mother." She hugged Mel tightly.

"You must be Mel," Beverly said when she reached the nurse's station.

"And you are Devin's mother," she replied.

"I'll leave you two to talk," Miriam said softly, and she walked away.

Mel extended her hand, but Beverly wrapped her arms around Mel instead. "Thank you so much," she whispered in Mel's ear. "Thank you for everything that you did for my son."

Mel hugged Beverly back. "I'm so sorry," she replied. "I'm sorry... for your... loss."

"Thank you," said Beverly, "but there's nothing to be sorry about.

You were wonderful to my son and you made his last days some of his happiest."

Mel pulled back and looked at Devin's mother, wearing a look of pure bewilderment on her face. "What?"

Beverly smiled. "I arrived just yesterday, shortly after you left work for the day. I spent three hours talking with Devin last night. Do you know who he talked about the entire time?"

Mel shrugged.

"You," she replied.

Mel swallowed hard, feeling a knot in her throat. "Me?"

"You," Beverly repeated. "He told me that he got really close to you. And that you were a very good friend to him."

Biting her lip, Mel nodded. "Not at first," she admitted, "but once I got to know him, I really liked him. A lot." She wiped her eyes. "I can't believe he's…"

"I know," Beverly said, pulling Mel back to hug her again. "Neither can I," she said.

"This is supposed to be the other way around," Mel said with a hint of a laugh. "Usually nurses are comforting and taking care of the family."

"Well let's just take care of each other, then," Beverly suggested.

Donna approached them, placing a hand gently on each of their shoulders. "Is there anything I can do? For either of you?"

Beverly shook her head. "I just need some rest," she said.

"I bet you do," Donna agreed. "Poor thing, you've been here all night."

"Well, I came straight here from the airport yesterday by cab, and hadn't planned to stay … but if one of you could help me find a hotel, and call me a cab —"

"You're welcome to stay with me," Mel offered. "My apartment is small, but I've got a guest room made up, and it would give you some privacy from all of the media."

Beverly's eyes brightened. "That's really kind of you to offer," she said. "Would I be imposing?"

"You wouldn't be imposing at all. It would be an honor to have you," Mel assured her.

Beverly considered it for a moment. "Okay then," she said with a nod. "I would really like to spend some time with you. I think it would help me feel closer to my son."

"So why don't the two of you go home," Donna suggested, looking at Mel. Then she turned to Beverly. "We'll call you at Mel's house when the autopsy is done and let you know what they've found."

Beverly nodded. "Thank you."

"I know this is a hard time to bring up a subject like this, but you're listed as Devin's next-of-kin in his medical record. We'll need to talk later today about what Devin's wishes were."

"Oh," Beverly said, dabbing her eyes with a tissue. She sniffled loudly. "We talked about it a few years ago after another injury on a movie set that could have been life-threatening. He said at the time that he wanted to be cremated and have his ashes scattered in the ocean."

Mel shuddered, thinking back to how she had created a journey to the bottom of the ocean for Devin just the day before.

Beverly sniffed loudly. "Cremation is not what I want as his mother, though. I want his body to be moved back home and buried next to his father in Florida."

Donna looked at her sympathetically. "I understand," she said. "I can't imagine what a tough decision it will be. I looked in Devin's medical record and he reported that he didn't have any kind of living will, and hadn't made any wishes known. He declared you as his next-of-kin, so the decision is yours to make."

"I'll have to do some thinking," Beverly said.

"Okay," Donna said. "We'll make those arrangements later today. Just go get some rest now."

"Should we get a security escort?" Mel asked. "I mean, since she's Devin's mom? What if someone knows who she is and won't leave us alone?"

"I'll walk with you," Brad volunteered. "The security guards up here aren't going to be able to break anytime soon. They've both been busy keeping unauthorized guests out of the unit, and I have a feeling it will only get worse as the day goes on."

As Mel and Brad led Beverly out into the parking lot and away from the hospital, Mel felt numb.

This can't be real. It has to be a dream. Devin was just fine yesterday. How could he have died?

Fortunately, none of the media circus seemed to make the connection that Beverly was Devin's mother, and no one bothered her. Just as they reached Mel's car, she glanced over at Beverly Ryan walking by her side, dabbing at her eyes with a crumbling tissue. Brad unlocked the passenger side door and held it for her as she climbed in, tucking her overnight bag on the floor between her feet. "Take care," he said to her. "I'm so sorry." He squeezed her hand gently before shutting the car door, then followed Mel to the driver's side and gave her a hug.

"Hang in there," he said.

"Thanks."

"You know where to find me if you need me, okay?"

"Sure."

This isn't how I was supposed to meet Beverly, Mel thought as she slipped into the driver's seat. *I was supposed to go into work today and find Devin in his bed and his mother sitting in a chair next to him, chatting away like they didn't have a care in the world. And Devin was supposed to introduce me to her, and then wait until I walked out of the room to tell her that she just met the woman of his dreams. And then Beverly was supposed to pull me aside and tease me about being her future daughter-in-law, and we'd have a good laugh or two and it would be our little inside joke...*

"Oh, Mel," Beverly said quite suddenly, "is this really happening? Did my baby really die?"

Mel looked at Devin's mother and slowly nodded. "Yes he did," she said. "And I'm so sorry, Beverly. I'm so very sorry."

***

"She got moved WHERE?" Brad asked.

"The ICU," Donna said. "Dr. Baylor was making rounds while

you stepped out to walk Mel and Beverly to the parking lot."

Brad shook his head. "What happened? Why did he move her?"

"He didn't like the way her lungs sounded," Donna said. "And she was non-responsive."

"Aughh!!!" Brad cried out. "That's what I told him the other day! Why did he wait until just now to move her?"

"Shhh," Donna cautioned him. "We need to mind what we say right now. We're getting a lot of attention from Devin Ryan passing away and you never know who could be lurking around the corner and listening in."

"I don't care," Brad said. "I told him yesterday she needed to be moved."

"I know you're frustrated," Donna said. "I can't tell you why the doctor made his decision, but right now we don't have any control over that. If you'd like to take a minute to go visit with Ms. Benson, then go ahead, but don't be long. I'm short one nurse on the floor now that Mel has gone home, and we've got three new post-op patients this morning. Can you be back in fifteen minutes?"

Brad nodded. "I'll be back in a few," he said.

On the elevator up to the ICU, Brad fought the urge to scream.

I should have been a better advocate for her, he scolded himself. *I should have called the doctor again yesterday. I had a bad feeling all day long about her, and she seemed to look worse every time I went into the room. Why didn't I call? Why didn't I insist?*

The elevator doors opened with a sharp *ding* onto the ICU, and Brad picked up the handset to the phone on the wall. It rang to the nurse's station.

"ICU, this is Andrea," answered a friendly voice.

"This is Brad from Med-Surg South. I just wanted to come see Amena Benson for a moment. She just moved up from our unit."

"Sure," Andrea said.

A loud buzzer sounded and Brad heard a sharp *click* as the doors to the ICU unlocked. Once inside, he washed his hands and went to the nurse's station. He found Andrea, a curly-haired brunette nurse that he guessed to be about his age, sitting behind a computer, peering studiously through her glasses at the data on the screen.

"Hi there," she said with a smile, looking up as he approached.

"So what's going on with her?" He asked.

"She's got a lot of fluid in her lungs," Andrea replied.

"Still coughing up blood?" Brad asked.

"Oh yes. And very short of breath."

Brad shook his head. "She was going downhill the other day. I thought she should have been admitted then. Is her daughter here?"

"Yes. She's in the consult room right now with Dr. Baylor." Andrea looked at him sympathetically. "You're welcome to go in to her room if you want to see her."

"Thanks. I will."

Andrea pointed to Amena's room and Brad stepped through the doorway. He paused to pray.

May there be peace in the world far and near, and may I bring peace to the person right here.

He approached Amena's bedside and wondered how it could be possible for her to look smaller and weaker than she had just a couple of days ago. Brad watched her tiny chest rise and fall too rapidly. He noticed that her nasal cannula had shifted and that the prongs were blowing air against her cheek instead of into her nose. He donned a pair of gloves and replaced it in her nostrils. His touch awakened her.

"Hello dear," she said weakly.

"Hi there," he replied.

"They took me away from you, Love. What ever will we do now?" She smiled weakly.

Brad couldn't help but smile. "It's good to hear your voice again." Brad paused for a moment. "You know, Amena, we've got plenty of patients getting discharged today on Med-Surg South, so why don't you get up out of that bed and come help me move them downstairs?" He joked.

She grinned, and her shoulders and chest vibrated slightly, as if she were laughing without her voice.

"You look sleepy," he said. "So I'm going to let you get some rest.

Is there anything I can do for you?"

But her eyelids had closed and she seemed to be resting again.

He stood to leave, tossed his gloves in the wastebasket, washed his hands and made it as far as the doorway.

"Brad?" She called out from behind him, so weakly that he almost didn't hear it. He turned.

"Yes?"

Her eyes were wide open, and she was smiling. "You're my angel," she said softly. "You're my peace."

Brad's heart began to thump so loudly that he could literally hear it. For a moment, all that he could do was just stand still, dumbfounded.

"What?" He finally asked.

But her eyes were already closed again, and she appeared to be sleeping soundly.

***

Mel awoke just as the sky had started to fade from a dusky blue to the black of night.

Where had the day gone? She wondered.

Suddenly, the memories came flooding back. She recalled going in to work that morning and getting the news that Devin had died...

Was it just a dream?

Then she remembered meeting Devin's mother, and decided that Beverly was too real for her to keep up any hopes of Devin's death being a bad dream. Beverly was real, all right, and was right there in Mel's apartment.

"Beverly... oh no!" Mel blurted out as she jumped out of bed, embarrassed for having been a bad host who had slumbered the day away. She smoothed the wrinkles out of her scrubs, which she had literally fallen asleep in, and stepped out of her bedroom.

Beverly was sitting on the sofa in the living room. Her eyes were puffy and red. She smiled when Mel entered the room, and held up an empty cardboard box that had once contained a full stack of fluffy white tissues.

"I owe you a box... or two," she said. "Sorry."

"Oh... please, don't worry about it," she said. "I'm so sorry I slept the day away. I laid down thinking I would nap for a couple of hours and before I knew it, I was waking up in the dark."

"It's okay," Beverly said. "You must have needed the rest. Devin told me that you've been working really hard. Long hours and extra shifts. I can't imagine how exhausted you must be, Mel."

Mel sat down on the sofa next to Beverly. "I'm just doing what I have to do for my family," she said.

"I know," Beverly nodded. "You're working yourself to the bone for your children, and your grandchild. What a heavy burden to bear, Mel."

"Devin told you all that about me?"

"Yes. And I met Jenny earlier today while you were sleeping. She made me lunch and we talked for a while. She's a lovely young woman, Mel. Very smart, and polite and thoughtful. If you don't mind me saying so, I think she's going to make a great mother," Beverly said.

"That's very kind of you," Mel said with a smile. "They were going to go spend the evening with their father and have dinner with him and his fiancée." She glanced at her watch. "Guess they left already."

"They left about thirty minutes ago," Beverly said. "Jenny didn't want to wake you."

Mel nodded. "Well what about you, Beverly? Were you able to nap in the guest room? Was it comfortable?"

"Yes, it was, and yes, I did," she replied. "Thank you so much for your hospitality. Honestly, I was dreading the thought of staying in a hotel all by myself." She looked at Mel again, and fresh tears were forming in her eyes. "The way that Devin spoke about you, Mel, you already felt like family to me. And had Devin pulled through, I feel strongly that you would have become a permanent fixture in his life. And in my life as well."

Mel blushed. "It's funny you'd say that. I felt the same way about you – that I knew you before I met you, and that we were almost... family."

"You've been wonderful to both my son, and to me," Beverly sniffled. "So as far as I'm concerned, we are family."

Mel smiled. "I'm honored to be a part of your family then." Then she frowned. "I just wish he were here," Mel said. "I still can't believe what happened. It doesn't seem real."

"I can't believe it either," Beverly said. "And the rest of the world won't believe it, not unless they see it. So I made some decisions this afternoon about what to do with Devin's body. And I'm going to need your help to carry them out."

Mel winced. She hadn't counted on being asked to help make Devin's final arrangements, and she didn't know if she would be able to handle going through with them. That would make his death definitively, unquestionably a reality, and Mel wasn't sure if she was ready to accept that or not. However, she felt like she owed it to Beverly. After all, they were family now.

"Okay," Mel agreed.

"First," Beverly said, pausing to catch a tear with the heel of her hand, "I'm going to have the local funeral home prepare Devin's body for a viewing. For myself, and for my brother and sister and their kids, who are on their way up from Florida, and for you and your colleagues on Med-Surg South that cared for him during his illness. Then, I'll work with his publicist to allow a select few members of the press to come in and have a no-cameras-allowed viewing, and we'll have a press conference to answer any questions about his death."

Mel nodded. So far, so good.

"And then, to honor Devin's wishes as best I can, he will be cremated and his ashes scattered in the ocean," she said, the pitch of her voice rising. She sniffled loudly and took several deep breaths before she could resume speaking. Mel reached out and took one of Beverly's hands into her own. "Or part of him will, anyway. The hospital called me about the autopsy today," she said tearfully. "As they suspected, he threw a clot which traveled from his broken leg to his heart, causing him to go into cardiac arrest."

"I'm so sorry," Mel said again, giving Beverly's hand a gentle squeeze.

Beverly nodded. "And then I made a bit of a non-traditional

request," she said. "I asked them if only his heart could be cremated. Since they had to take it out of him…"

"Oh?" Mel asked.

"And they agreed to help make the arrangements. I want to leave his heart here in Dogwood with you, Mel. It belongs to you, anyway."

Mel bit her lip and wiped her eyes.

"And I want to ask you to please take the ashes from my son's heart and scatter them across the ocean, as he wished. Would you be willing to do that?"

"Of course," Mel said. "Of course I will."

"The rest of his body – everything but the heart – will go home with me, and will be laid to rest next to his father. That may not be the way that Devin planned it, but it's the decision that I'm making for him."

"I understand."

"It's very important to me that he be with his father now. He never knew him when he was alive."

Nodding, Mel looked at Beverly. "I know. Devin told me about that."

"Did he mention how his father died?"

Shaking her head from side to side, Mel looked away. "No, he didn't." The raw ache in her heart dug even deeper. Beverly was a widow who lost her only son. Mel couldn't even begin to imagine how much pain she was feeling at the moment.

"I want to tell you that story, if you don't mind," Beverly said.

"Of course I don't mind. I'm all ears."

Beverly sat quietly for another moment. Mel didn't rush her. When she was ready, she spoke.

"Devin's father was a good man. Joseph was my high school sweetheart. We both finished our senior year, and then we got married. Neither of us went to college. I got pregnant two months after our wedding, and he went to work at a textile mill while I stayed at home and got ready for Devin to arrive. It was a wonderful time in our lives, Mel. He and I were inseparable. Up until that point, I'd never been happier in my life."

"It sounds wonderful," she said, trying desperately not to think about her own years of wedded bliss with Bruce, and the sting that followed when her marriage was taken away from her. For the first time, she considered that losing a husband to death was probably the only thing more painful than losing a husband to divorce.

"The month before I was due to deliver, my sister decided to throw a baby shower for me," Beverly continued. "She lived three hours away, so we left home about noon that day. It was a surprise, of course. I thought we were just going for a visit, but Joseph and my sister had been scheming and planning, and when we arrived, all of our friends and family were there to greet me. There were baby gifts from wall to wall, and food as far as the eye could see... they even made blue punch, can you imagine? We didn't even know that we were having a boy. My sister said she just had a feeling."

Mel chuckled softly. "Smart sister," she said.

Beverly nodded and continued. "We packed everything up in the car after the shower. I wanted to stay longer, but Joseph wanted us to get home before it got too dark. So we started home. We were only thirty minutes from our house. When a driver in a truck in the opposite lane fell asleep at the wheel. He swerved into our lane. Joseph cut the wheel to the right, trying to take us onto the shoulder to avoid getting hit. There just wasn't enough time. The truck hit us, and our car rolled over."

Mel closed her eyes. She imagined the two vehicles slamming together, the squealing tires, and the smell of burning rubber on asphalt.

"It happened so fast. Thinking back, I barely remember it. I think I lost consciousness shortly after it happened, because I don't remember anything else until I arrived at the hospital."

"What about the baby?" Mel felt foolish for asking, already knowing the answer; that Devin had survived without any obvious or enduring harm. Still, she knew there was more to the story.

Beverly smiled. "Devin was born that night," she said. "About a month early. The trauma I suffered from the wreck made me go into labor, and once he started making his way out, there was no stopping him. The next thing I remember was being strapped down on a stretcher, with the paramedics rushing me into the hospital and nurses and doctors swarming around me to take over. I heard all of them talking about my cuts and contusions and broken bones, but I couldn't feel any of that. All that I could feel were the contractions. They were strong and hard, and so close together that I knew it wouldn't be long."

"That must have been so hard, delivering your baby and knowing that you had just lost your husband," Mel said softly, blinking to break up the tears filling her eyes.

"But that wasn't the case at all," Beverly said with excitement. "He was there with me, Mel. Once they moved me into the delivery room, he was there by my side. He held my hand, wiped the sweat from my forehead, and he coached me through the contractions. He talked me through the entire thing. And when I gave birth, the doctor put him in my arms and congratulated me on my baby boy. At that point I passed out, I think."

"So what happened next?" Mel was on the edge of the seat, wringing her hands nervously.

"I slept for several days, they said. When I awoke, I had a cast on one leg, my arm in a sling, stitches all over my body, and shortly after, a baby in my arms. I asked for Joseph, and I was told that he had died in the wreck. I told them they were mistaken, and I shared with them how he'd been right by my side while I was giving birth. They told me that was impossible. When the truck hit us, it broke Joseph's neck and killed him instantly. He was thrown from the vehicle. In fact, he had been thrown so far that they searched for hours to find him. I went to the hospital in the ambulance alone."

A chill passed through Mel's spine. "Wow," was all that she could muster.

"I insisted that Joseph had been there with me the whole time. I told everyone how wonderful he had been during the birth of his son. You know what they told me, Mel? They said that I either dreamed or imagined it. They said that the pain medication could have caused me to hallucinate. They said that what I saw and heard and felt when Joseph was there, wasn't real."

Mel shook her head, bewildered.

"After everything that happened that night, Mel, I don't think that anyone had the right to tell me what was real and what wasn't."

Mel blinked several times, and waited for Beverly to continue.

"I know Joseph was there with me when Devin was born. No one can ever take that away from me. His body may have been lying dead on the side of the road, but he was with me. Something happened that night that was truly divine. Divine. And when they asked me for a name for my baby, that's the word that was in my mind. I played around with the letters and I came up with Devin. With an "i" left over."

"Devin and I," Mel said.

"Exactly," she said. "That divine event, whatever it was, and however it happened, it was just for Devin and I. No one else in the world would ever be able to understand or believe our own little miracle."

"That's... incredible," Mel whispered. The nurse in her knew that pain medication, hallucinations and dreams were the more likely explanation, as Beverly's caregivers had told her at the time. But Beverly's sincerity of her belief in what happened the night that Joseph died and Devin was born was as solid as a rock.

"I know what you must be thinking," Beverly said, obviously sensing Mel's discomfort with her story. "And you don't have to believe me. It's okay. It would be quite a leap to trust in something that outrageous. But it was real, Mel. It really happened."

Mel smiled. "I believe that you believe it," she said. "And that's real enough for me."

Beverly shook her head. "I don't just believe in it, Mel. I know it."

Mel arched her eyebrows curiously. "Believing... knowing... how are they different?"

"Believing takes work. It takes convincing yourself of the truth. Believing means that even though you have doubts lurking in your mind, you have faith that is even stronger. And that's a very good thing. We all need something to believe in. But when you know something, Mel, there's no work required, and there are no doubts. Ever."

Mel nodded, processing Beverly's explanation.

"That's what it means to know. It's whatever is real to you, Mel, even in the absence of proof for others. It's a wisdom that comes from within."

"I understand... I think," Mel said.

"Of course you do. Do you know for certain that tomorrow will come, or do you just believe?"

Mel thought for a moment. "I guess I believe that tomorrow will come. I don't have many reasons not to. I believe that I'll wake up tomorrow, and that the earth will be spinning, and we'll all live to see another day. I don't know for sure, and I can't prove it, but I have faith that it will happen. I believe in tomorrow."

Beverly nodded. "Now tell me, do you love Jenny and Michael?'

"Yes. With all my heart."

"And do you believe that you love them? Or do you know that you love them?"

"I *know* I love my children," Mel said, without hesitation. "I couldn't prove it to you or anyone else, but I don't need to. It's so real to me that I know for sure."

"Then you get it," Beverly said. "And I feel the same way. I know I love my son. And I know that wherever he is right now, he's with my Joseph, and somehow, both of them will always be with me. Even if I can't see them or hear them or touch them. I'm going to miss that part of them, Mel. The part of them that I could see and hear and touch and hold. That part of them is gone, and I have some wonderful memories to soothe the ache of losing that. But everything else about them is still here, still very much alive, and always will be. And knowing that is one of two things that is giving me the strength to get through this."

"What's the other?"

Beverly smiled. "You." She reached out her arms, and Mel fell into them. They wept and hugged each other for a long time.

"You fell in love with my boy, didn't you, Mel?"

Mel sniffled loudly. "I'm afraid I did."

"I knew that too," Beverly said.

***

"Code Blue, ICU, Code Blue, ICU." The voice on the hospital-wide loudspeaker spoke loudly, and with urgency.

Brad shot up out of his seat in the cafeteria, abandoning the grilled cheese sandwich and potato chips that he had purchased for his late lunch.

Please, not Amena... please, not her!

He pumped his arms by his side as he raced for the elevator. His heart pounded as he dashed through the open doors and pressed the button to the ICU floor. The elevator doors slid shut, and he began the slow ascent to the Intensive Care Unit.

"Come on, COME ON!" He cried out, jabbing his index finger on the floor button, as if it would make the elevator go faster. He felt jittery from the adrenaline rushing through his body.

Please! He cried out on his mind. *If there is a Higher Power out there... Jesus, Buddha, Mohammad, whoever... I don't care! Please don't take her right now!*

He closed his eyes and saw Grandmother Lillian in her casket again. The memory of her face was as fresh as if he'd seen her just yesterday. Even with her eyes closed, she bore a striking resemblance to Amena Benson.

Not Amena too. Not now. Please. PLEASE!

The elevator door opened, and Brad rushed to the phone on the wall outside of the ICU. He picked up the handset and waited while it rang. And rang, and rang, and rang, and rang.

And rang some more. He hung it up and went to the door, pounding on it with his fists.

"It's Brad from Med-Surg South," he cried out. "Andrea... anyone... let me in, please!"

As he waited, he could hear his blood pulsing in his ears.

"Anyone... please!" Even as he pounded on the door again, he realized that most, if not all of the ICU staff were tied up working the code, and that it would likely be impossible for him to pass through the doors until the code was over.

"Is there a problem?" A deep male voice asked from behind him.

Brad whirled around and found himself face to face with Dr. Baylor.

"Let me in," he demanded.

"I don't think so," Dr. Baylor said sharply. "You need to calm down. They're working a code in there—"

"Which is exactly why I need to go in. My friend is in there and I need to know that it's not her." Brad spoke quickly and loudly.

Dr. Baylor advanced a step toward him. "You need to get yourself under control. I can't let you in there. Not like this."

Brad felt as if he could throw flames from his mouth. "If it's her," he began, "If it's Amena Benson, then you better get in there and save her! I called you the other day and told you that she needed to be moved to the ICU! Why did you wait?" He threw up his hands in frustration.

"Calm down and lower your tone of voice," Dr. Baylor said firmly, "or I'll call security. Go back to your unit and I'll call you as soon as I have news about Ms. Benson. I'm not letting you into the ICU."

Just what I need, Brad thought. *To get in trouble for blowing up at a doctor.*

Angrily, he rushed down the hall to the elevator once again.

***

Back at Med Surg South, Brad parked himself in a chair at the nurse's station and drummed his fingers on the desk, waiting for Dr. Baylor's call. His heart pounded away in his chest.

Ten minutes later, the phone rang.

"Med-Surg South, Brad speaking."

"It's Dr. Baylor."

"And?"

There was a brief pause on the other end of the line. "I'm very sorry. Ms. Benson was the patient who coded and we were not able to resuscitate her."

Brad's thumping heart suddenly felt as if it were going to explode. "It's your fault," he said, then hung up the phone, almost slamming it down.

"Whoa," Donna said, her eyes growing wide as she approached the nurse's station. "What's going on here?"

Sinking his head into his hands, Brad took a deep breath. "She died," he said. "The code in the ICU… that was Ms. Benson."

"Oh… Brad, Honey, I'm so sorry…" Donna rolled up a chair next to him and sat down, placing a caring hand on his shoulder. "I'm so very sorry."

"Two of our patients in one day," Brad sighed. "I think we've set some kind of a new record here, haven't we?" He looked up, shaking his head.

"Honey, it's not your fault," Donna consoled him. "You did everything you could for her."

"I know it's not my fault," Brad snapped. "It's Dr. Baylor's fault. He should have admitted her when I told him to. She was going downhill. I could see it, and I told him. But he didn't listen."

Donna looked at him with empathy. "Sometimes doctors make tough decisions," she said.

"Sometimes they even make the wrong decisions," Brad retorted.

"I know," Donna said. "And I know that as nurses we often feel like there has to be someone to blame for a death, whether it's ourselves, or someone else, but let's not get caught in that trap right now, Brad. And I'd be glad to talk with Dr. Baylor about why he didn't admit her earlier. There's probably a good reason why. But in the meantime, there's nothing we can do now. It must have been her time to go."

"Oh… don't do that, Donna. Don't use the 'Jesus calls his little children home when it's their time' line on me." He shook his head grimly. "It wasn't her time. And this is bull. She just had pneumonia. Not cancer or renal failure, or anything else terminal. She could have been helped. She could have lived another five or ten years."

"I'm sorry, Brad. That's all I know to tell you right now. That, and you are too upset to be here right now. You should clock out and go home."

He shook his head angrily as he rose to leave. "It's not fair," he said. "She was a good person. She didn't deserve this."

Chapter 13
Monday

Mel waved at Brad from across the employee parking deck. "Hey stranger," she called out. She spoke loudly, but without enthusiasm. Her tone suggested that she was still tired.

He crossed several rows of cars to meet her, forcing a polite smile as he did so. Mel stretched out her arms as he approached, and hugged him when he reached her.

"How are you doing?" She asked.

"Probably about as well as you are."

"Yeah. I'm really sorry about Ms. Benson."

"And I'm sorry about Devin. How are you?"

Mel sighed deeply. "I'm okay, I guess. I thought about stopping by over the weekend to see how you were doing, but I was tied up helping Devin's mom make arrangements on Saturday. I dropped her off at the airport early yesterday morning, and then I went home and went back to bed. I slept through yesterday. I don't know if I'm depressed or if all of my fatigue has finally caught up with me. Or maybe it's a combination of both."

"Probably both," Brad said, as they turned toward the parking deck exit and began to make their way to the employee entrance of the hospital. "And you're grieving too. You probably shouldn't even be at work today."

"I can't afford to miss any days. I'm saving up my vacation time for when Jenny delivers the baby. And speaking of grieving, so are you," Mel scolded. "How come you're working today?"

"What else am I supposed to do?" Brad asked.

"Grieve," Mel responded. "You were close to Ms. Benson."

"Not that close," he said. "And yeah, I'm sad over the whole thing, but I'm not going to put my life on hold. I can't afford to take any days off either. I'm back to one income without Sue around to help me pay the bills, and I'm saving up my vacation time for the summer. Miriam and I have talked about going out to the beach for a week and joining one of those fishing expedition groups."

"Really?" Mel asked, smiling and nudging him playfully in the side. "So now that Sue is gone, is Miriam your new girlfriend? Or should I be jealous – has she replaced me as your best friend at work?"

"Come on. You know it's nothing like that," Brad grinned sheepishly. "Miriam and I have sort of been hanging out lately. Talking a lot. And fishing. I think it's helping me process everything that's going on right now in my life. She's actually a really good person to talk to."

Mel smiled. "Well, good," she said. "I'm glad that you're talking to somebody. I was feeling bad all this time, thinking that I wasn't being much of a best friend. We haven't talked in so long."

"Don't feel bad. It goes both ways. I haven't been around for you much, either. And I was worried that Devin was going to replace me as your new best bud."

Mel shrugged. "Well, he and I got close, but we both know how that turned out. So let's get back on track. How about we get lunch together in the cafeteria today?"

"Well," Brad began, "I sort of have other plans for today. How about tomorrow?"

"Deal," Mel replied.

They walked in silence for a little while.

"So you and Miriam have been talking?" Mel asked. "What about?"

"Well… everything. Sue leaving me. And her losing Homer. And fishing. And dogs. And all kinds of other stuff."

"I have to admit, I'm a little bit jealous," Mel joked. "What does Miriam have that I don't?"

Brad exhaled loudly. "It's not like that, Mel. You know you're my best friend. But sometimes Miriam is just easier to talk to."

Mel was taken aback. "How so?"

"She doesn't hate men, for one," Brad said.

"Neither do I."

"Yeah you do. It's hard for me to listen to you spout off about what a scumbag Bruce was, and how you'll never trust another man for the rest of your life, and be the man on the other end of the conversation just trying to be a friend to you."

Ouch, Mel thought to herself. *Brad has a point.*

"Touché," she said. "I'm sorry. I didn't realize how I was coming across. I never meant to hurt your feelings. I do trust you, Brad. I hope you know that."

"Yeah," he said. "I know. And I hope you know that I didn't mean anything against you by confiding in Miriam about things. She's just been really easy to talk to."

"It's okay," Mel said, touching his arm. "I understand. We all need friends. Everyone needs somebody to tell things to, when life gets tough. And if you're lucky, you have more than one."

"Then I'm lucky," Brad said, as he badged in and walked through the employee entrance.

"We both are," Mel said, swiping her own badge and following him through the open door.

***

At lunchtime, Brad wandered up to the ICU. He picked up the telephone mounted on the wall. Andrea answered it before he even heard a ring.

"ICU, this is Andrea."

"Hi. It's Brad from Med-Surg South."

The buzzer sounded. Brad hung up the phone and stepped

through the doors to the unit.

At the nurse's station, Andrea rose from a seated position and looked at him sympathetically as he walked toward her. "Hi," she said.

"Hey," he responded.

Andrea pushed her glasses up on her nose and looked away nervously for a second. Brushing a stray lock of hair from her forehead and tucking it behind her ear, she looked back up at Brad. "I'm... I'm really sorry," she said. "About Ms. Benson. We did everything that we could."

Brad nodded. "I know," he said softly. "I was wondering if you might be free for lunch today. I'm on my way down to the cafeteria and I was going to see if you'd like to join me. My treat."

Andrea blushed. "Oh," she said, smiling. "Um... yeah. Okay. Sure. Let me just let everyone else know that I'm stepping out, because I normally go to lunch around two o'clock." She disappeared around the bend of the nurse's station for a moment, and then returned. "Ready," she announced.

In the cafeteria, Brad picked out a cheeseburger and potato chips for his lunch. Andrea fixed a small salad and topped it with chickpeas and a vinaigrette dressing. They found a seat near a window, where sunlight poured through. Window seats were usually the coveted spots in the cafeteria, as they offered a view of the beautifully landscaped front lawn of the hospital, with lush floral blooms of every kind, and Dogwood trees scattered throughout. Normally, it was nice scenery, but on this particular day, it was crowded with journalists and camera crews who were still reporting on Devin's death, and strangers who had arrived on the scene early for the candlelight vigil to be held later that night.

"I'm ready for all those media types to pack up and move on," Andrea said, glancing out the window.

"You and me both," Brad agreed before biting into his cheeseburger.

"Yeah." Andrea looked down and poked at her salad with a plastic fork. "Let the poor guy rest in peace, right?"

Nodding, Brad put his burger down for a moment. "But speaking of resting in peace, I was hoping you could tell me about Amena Benson. Do you know what happened? Why did she code?"

Andrea's face melted into a look of distress. "She had all of this fluid in her lungs," she began.

"Yeah, I knew that."

"Dr. Baylor had her on a diuretic, but I guess it wasn't enough." Andrea blinked several times and took a deep breath. "I worked the code," she said. "And we tried so hard. We did everything that we could. I swear we did. She was Dr. Putnam's mother-in-law, you know. None of us wanted to have to tell him that we had lost her."

Brad nodded. "I know it must have been hard."

Andrea cocked an eyebrow. "How did you know her?" She asked. "Was she family?"

"No. She was just a friend. She volunteered here at Dogwood. That's how I knew her. That's how we all knew her."

"Oh," Andrea said. "I'm new. I've only been here for two months. I hadn't met her prior to her being admitted to our unit."

"Where did you work before coming here?" Brad asked.

"At a hospital in Virginia. I'm from Dogwood originally, but moved to Virginia with my husband five years ago. Only that didn't last long. We just finalized our divorce, and I came back home to live with my mom and dad."

Brad frowned. "Sorry to hear that."

She waved her hand in the air dismissively. "It's okay," she said. "You know what people say... what doesn't kill us only makes us stronger."

"Right," he nodded. "So you were an ICU nurse in Virginia too?"

"Yeah. I've worked in Emergency, ICU and Critical Care."

"Thrill seeker," he smiled. "You like living on the edge?"

Andrea shook her head. "It's not about thrills. I just like being able to help people."

"But you can't save them all," Brad insisted. "I was a medic in the Navy, and a paramedic prior to becoming a nurse. I've seen enough death and tragedy to last a lifetime. And I bet you have too."

"Of course I have. But I never said that I do this to 'save' lives. I said 'help.' I like being able to help people in crisis."

Brad sat silently for a moment, chewing on his lunch and thinking through Andrea's words. "So, what's the difference?"

"The difference is, you don't have to save someone's life to help them. Sometimes helping a person means that you're providing them comfort while they're preparing for death. Sometimes it means you help them find peace so that they can die without regrets or sorrow. Sometimes you're helping them just by fighting for their life, and doing everything that you can to save them. I've seen a lot of people in Emergency and ICU and Critical Care that the rest of the world didn't care about anymore. Like teenage runaways who were living on the street. Criminals with a shady past. Elderly people who had basically been abandoned by their families after being admitted to a nursing home. People that the rest of the world gave up on. I fought for them. We all did. We fought to keep them alive, and in the process of doing so, we showed them that their lives had worth and meaning. You don't fight for something if it's worth nothing."

Brad sat quietly. He peered over the rims of Andrea's glasses, looking into her blue eyes.

"And we fought hard for Ms. Benson," Andrea continued. "But we still couldn't save her. I'm sorry, Brad."

Nodding slightly, he sank back into his chair. "Did she suffer?"

"I had no reason to believe that she did. One minute, she was lying in bed, struggling to breathe, and the next thing I know, she just stopped. And then her heart stopped. The only discomfort that I ever saw in Ms. Benson was in her struggle to keep breathing and to stay alive. When she went, it was effortless. She didn't fight it at all. To me, it seemed peaceful."

He sat silently for a moment. "Was she alone before she went? Or was her daughter there?"

Andrea leaned forward slightly. "Cassandra was there when she stopped breathing. And prior to that, Dr. Putnam came and sat with her for a while, and they both held her hands. And she had some visitors earlier in the day. A group of elderly ladies. Friends, I suppose. And then a couple with young children. Family, I'm sure. And you. I remember that you came to visit her. But to answer your question, no. She was not alone at any point."

Brad nodded. "Okay," he said softly, and then added, "I didn't get to tell her goodbye."

Andrea put down her fork and stared at him across the table. "It's not too late. Her funeral is tomorrow. And the family is receiving visitors tonight at the funeral home. Why don't you go to one or the other? Maybe it would give you some peace about the situation."

He arched an eyebrow. "Peace?"

"Peace," she echoed, with a nod.

***

First shift came and went in the blink of an eye. Mel was exhausted. She made her way to the employee exit and badged out. When she opened the door, she was amazed at the sight. Hundreds, if not thousands of flickering candles sprinkled across the lawn of Dogwood Regional Medical; some on the ground and some in the hands of people, providing a sharp contrast of light against the dimming horizon. Floral bouquets lined the ground. Posters and pictures of Devin Ryan were everywhere. But all eyes fixed on where she stood in the doorway, as they probably did each time any employee exited the building.

Cameras were rolling, she was sure. But she could take it no longer.

"What's wrong with you people?" Mel cried out at the top of her lungs. "Who do you think you are? Moping around with your candles and flowers like you actually lost someone... like you actually knew him!"

A flood of lights suddenly illuminated the lawn. A small crowd of reporters began to make their way toward her, each intent on being the first to get live footage of the crazy lady losing her cool at Devin Ryan's memorial site. The non-media mourners simply looked at her curiously.

"None of you knew him! None of you knew anything about him!" Mel scolded them, screaming loud enough for all to hear. "All you care about is Devin Ryan, the hotshot movie star. Well, let me tell you, folks, you know nothing about Devin Ryan, the human being. And he was a good, kind man. He didn't deserve to die. And he certainly doesn't deserve all of you out here, prancing around like it's some kind of media circus and making a mockery of his memory!"

It became so quiet, one could hear a pin drop.

Tears were pouring down Mel's cheeks. "Why don't you all just go home? Why can't you let him rest? Just leave him alone. Leave him ALONE!"

Heads began to turn as people looked to each other in the crowd, the obvious question burning in their minds: Should we listen to this livid, shouting woman and leave, or just ignore her?

A few people stirred as if they planned to move, but no one actually packed up their mourning paraphernalia and started walking.

"Amazing," Mel muttered. "You people are amazing."

Mel made her way down the steps and followed the footpath to the employee parking deck. She watched the faces of the people lining the path as she walked by them. Looks of confusion and concern were etched into their faces.

Stupid media hounds, Hollywood types, local wannabes, all of you losers... go get a life of your own and quit fixating on someone else's! She wanted to scream.

Then she stopped short.

A little boy stepped into her path, almost colliding with her. Mel would have knocked him over and kept moving, had she not recognized his face.

She'd seen him somewhere before. He was at least five years old, possibly six, but definitely no older than seven. Huge glasses, teeth too big for the rest of his mouth, hair curled into tight corkscrews. He was so awkward looking that he was adorable.

He removed his glasses and dragged a hand across his face to wipe the tears that were pouring down his face.

"Excuse me," he said, "Do you know Devin Ryan?"

Mel shrugged. "No comment," she said absentmindedly.

Then, she realized where she had seen the child before. He was the same little boy who had appeared on the newscast announcing Devin's arrival in Dogwood. The very newscast that she had watched only days ago with Jenny. It seemed like an eternity had passed since then.

"Did you go in his room?" The little boy asked. "Were you one of his nurses?"

"I…. I can't comment on that," Mel said.

"Do you know if he got my card? I just want to know if he got my card."

"I'm sure that he got a lot of cards and letters …"

"Do you know if he got mine? My name is Justin Creech, and I sent a card that had a picture of a duck in a wheelchair. And I wrote a message inside…I just didn't know if he would read it or not, since I'm just a kid…"

Mel's heart leaped. She knelt down on one knee so that she was face to face with the boy.

"Devin loved your card. And he loved kids."

And he loved me, Mel thought to herself, biting her lip and trying not to cry. *He loved me, and now he's gone.*

"He was my hero," Justin said.

"He was a lot of people's hero, sweetheart," Mel whispered. "He certainly was mine." She stood up and turned all the way around, looking at the crowd of people surrounding her. She felt ashamed for having unleashed her rage on these poor strangers.

Mel began to cry. *Devin didn't just belong to me, or to Med-Surg South, or to Beverly, or to the media. He meant something to everyone here. And they have every right to grieve his loss.*

All eyes were still on her. "I'm sorry, everyone… I'm sorry," Mel said.

She ran to her car as fast as she could, never looking back, knowing that she wouldn't be able to see anyway through her tears.

***

Brad rushed home to change out of his scrubs into a suit and tie, and dashed across town to the funeral home. His plan was simple – get through the door, say goodbye to Amena, and get out. He was tired and wasn't in the mood to linger and make small talk with strangers.

When he walked through the door, a gray-haired, sweet-faced lady directed Brad to sign the guest registry. Glancing at the other names on the page, he spotted one that caught his attention – Andrea Pecachek. He didn't know the last name of Andrea from ICU, but had a strong suspicion that it was her.

He followed a crowd of other visitors down a long hallway, until he saw a marquee reading "Benson Family" pointing toward a large parlor. When he entered, there were several familiar faces from Dogwood Regional Medical Center. Several of the other volunteers that Amena had worked with were there, as were many of the nurses and other employees of Dogwood who had grown close to her. Many of the physicians and their spouses had come to give their condolences to Dr. Putnam and Cassandra. But Brad was looking for one face in particular, and quickly found it.

Andrea looked a lot different minus the raspberry-colored scrubs, white sneakers, smart-looking glasses and tousled ponytail, the typical look that Brad had come to associate with her. She was wearing a fitted black dress and high heels, and her curly hair hung just below her shoulders. When her ocean-blue eyes met Brad's from across the room, she smiled.

Wow, he thought. *She's really quite pretty.*

Andrea crossed the room to greet him. "Hi Brad."

"Hey," he said. "How long have you been here?"

"Just a few minutes. I've been chatting with some of the family members. Everyone's waiting for them to open the doors to the other room so we can go in and view her body. Right now it's just immediate family with her." She pointed to the set of double doors.

Brad nodded. "I'm not staying for long. Not a huge fan of this kind of stuff. I just came to say goodbye and then I'm out of here."

"Same here. I would stay longer but I put in a twelve hour shift today and I've got another one coming up tomorrow. I'm tired."

"Are you going to the funeral tomorrow?"

"Probably not," she shook her head. "We've got one nurse out on maternity leave right now, and another on vacation. It will be impossible to get away. What about you?"

"Yeah. I think I'm going."

The doors to the viewing room opened, and the crowd of visitors lined up to make their way in. The line moved quickly, and Brad and Andrea were through the doors before they knew it. Cassandra Putnam was first in the line to receive condolences and thank visitors for coming. She hugged both of the nurses and thanked them for all that they did for her mother. Brad shook hands with the rest of the family and expressed his sorrow, and before he knew it, he was standing over Amena's casket.

She was wearing a pretty pink suit and a white blouse with a ruffled collar. Her silvery white hair framed her face in neat, tight curls, and her cheeks seemed full again. There were a few telltale smudges of poorly blended cosmetic foundation at the base of her neck and her hairline, but otherwise, she looked well. As if she were just sleeping. And she still looked so much like Grandma Lillian.

Brad took a deep breath and reached into the casket, wrapping his hand around hers. "It's been a privilege knowing you, Amena," he said in almost a whisper. "I'm going to miss seeing you around. Wherever you are now, I hope that you've found peace. And if it's not too much to ask... send some my way, will you? My heart is broken." He did his best to hold back tears. "Goodbye, my friend."

Brad made his way back to the entrance of the funeral home and waited for Andrea to appear. He held the door for her and they made their way to the parking lot together.

"I'm glad we ran into each other," Brad said.

"Me too."

He walked her to her car and held the driver's side door open for her.

"Hey, have you eaten dinner?" She asked.

"Not yet."

"Me neither." She hesitated for a second. "Well... would you like to go get something to eat?"

Brad wasn't sure about having dinner with Andrea. She was really nice. And quite attractive, and obviously interested in him. But now wasn't the right time. There were three other women in his thoughts — Amena, Grandma Lillian and Sue. And it wouldn't be fair to Andrea to take her to dinner, knowing that she would be the last thing on his mind.

"I'm sorry," I can't," Brad apologized. "Not tonight, anyway. But

I'd love to have dinner with you some other time."

Andrea looked a little disappointed at first, and then smiled. "That's fine. Whenever you're ready Brad." She pulled a piece of paper from her purse, wrote down her phone number and handed it to him. "Call me sometime. Or just drop by the ICU."

"I will," he promised, as he began to make his way to his own car.

"Hey Brad?" Andrea called out to him.

He turned to her.

"You don't have to go through this alone," she said. "I'm not saying it has to be me… but talk to someone. You seem a lot quieter than you normally are."

He looked at her strangely. "What do you mean 'quieter than I normally am?' We just met a few days ago."

She smiled. "I know we just met, but I've seen you …. you know… walking through the halls and in the cafeteria. You're always talking and laughing and hanging out with the other nurses from your unit. You just seem so quiet lately. I like you the other way."

He laughed. "It sounds like you have been watching me for a while."

She covered her face with her hands and laughed softly. "I totally just told on myself, I guess."

"Stalker," he joked.

"Hey," she said, feigning a wounded look, "I am not. I'm just… interested."

Brad smiled. "I'm just kidding. And I'm flattered. And I'm interested too."

Andrea blushed and covered her smile with her hand.

"I just need some time… if that's okay."

"I understand. Take your time," Andrea said.

They waved goodbye as Brad climbed into his car and started the engine. He tucked the scrap of paper with Andrea's number on it into his pants pocket. Then he pulled it back out and slid it into his wallet, trusting that it would be safer there. And in doing so, he came across a picture of Sue. Beautiful, blonde, smiling Sue, who still reigned over his heart, who he still couldn't believe was gone.

Brad glanced around the parking lot a few times, and when he was sure that no one else was there, he rested his forehead on the steering wheel and cried for a very long time.

Chapter 14
Tuesday

Mel dried her eyes in the rearview mirror, blotting away a mascara smudge. Then she stepped out of her car in the employee parking deck and made her way to the hospital.

She had dreamed about Devin last night. What a wonderful dream. He had shown up on Mel's doorstep and taken her into his arms, then hugged her and kissed her.

She wept on his shoulder.

"Devin, I thought you were dead! Don't ever scare me like that again!"

"I'm here now, my beautiful girl. Everything is going to be okay," he had told her.

When she awoke, the dream was still lingering, still teasing her with an alternate ending to her and Devin's story. She curled up on her side, smiling and waiting for Devin to come and wrap his arms around her. She remembered that he had found his way to her apartment and that he was inside. She just wasn't sure where he was at the moment… maybe he was in the kitchen making her breakfast…

And then, very abruptly, reality slapped her in the face and the dream was over.

This is not fair. This is not fair. This is not fair. The four words became her mantra.

***

At work, Mel went through the motions and cared for her patients in autopilot mode, without much thought or feeling.

Her numbness quickly turned into embarrassment when Janice Murphy, the Director of Public Relations showed up on Med-Surg South and requested an impromptu meeting with her.

She steered Mel into the break room and placed the daily news paper in front of her. Mel could feel her eyes nearly bulge out of her skull when she saw her picture on the front page. It had been taken the night before, when she yelled at the visitors on the front lawn of the hospital.

"Angry Nurse Causes Uproar at Devin Ryan Memorial Site" was the headline.

Mel covered her face with her hands. "Oh my God, Janice, I'm so sorry."

Janice took a deep breath. "Well, we've received some interesting phone calls about it today, and our response to everyone is that the loss of Devin Ryan was a very stressful event for you, and we're asking for compassion and understanding."

"I'm sorry, I really am," Mel said, as she wailed into her cupped hands.

"I know this is tough," Janice said. "I was a Med-Surg nurse for fourteen years. I lost my share of patients too. But Mel, you need to get over this, and fast."

She met Janice's eyes with her own. "I've lost patients before too," she explained. "But this was different. Devin and I got very close. We were—"

"In love, yes, I've heard. And I'm truly sorry about the way this ended. But come on, Mel. You only knew him for what... a week? How close could you really get to somebody in a week's time? We lost one of our volunteers this week, Amena Benson—"

"Who was one of our patients also," Mel said. "I know."

"There are a lot of people in this hospital who are very sad about that, and I'm sure that there were bonds that ran even deeper between Amena and the employees and other volunteers of this hospital than the attachment you had to Devin. But they're getting on with their lives. You can't mope and mourn forever. You work in a hospital, for crying out loud, and people are going to die. If you can't handle that, then maybe you should consider a career change."

Mel felt as if she had been slapped in the face. "You have no right to say that to me," she said. "What happened to the compassion and understanding? You're asking everyone else to grant me that, but you're saying that I'm not entitled to it from you?"

Janice frowned. "I am being compassionate and understanding," she said. "I've spent all day cleaning up your mess. I could have had you written up, but I didn't. I'm trying to be nice, Mel, and I'm hoping we can just let this go. But I'm letting you know now, you need to get over it."

Mel took a deep breath and blotted her eyes again. "Okay," she said. "I'll do the best I can."

Janice tried to look sympathetic. "I am sorry for your loss," she said. "Or losses, rather."

"Thank you," Mel said softly.

***

Halfway through the day, Donna pulled Mel into her office. "You don't look so good, Honey. It would be okay if you wanted to take a day off. You know that, don't you?"

Mel nodded. "It's not going to do me any good. It's better for me to be here. It gives me something to do. If I'm at home, I won't be doing anything but lying in bed and crying."

Donna touched her hand. "Maybe that's what you need to be doing," she said. "Right now your mind is elsewhere, that's very clear. And that scares me a little bit because zombies don't make good nurses. That critical thinking stuff that's part of your job… that's something you have to take seriously, you know."

Mel smiled. "I know. And if I knew how to snap out of this, I would. But I just can't right now."

"Do you want to talk about it?"

Mel shook her head no.

"Well, we need to do something for you, Mel. I'm really concerned about you."

Mel nodded. "Let me go talk to David," she said. "He's been a big help in the past. I've had some questions that I think he could probably answer for me, and if he could, it would help me find some peace."

"That sounds like a good idea," Donna said. "Why don't you go ahead and see if you can catch him now?"

"I will."

"Good. And Mel, how is Brad? Have you talked to him lately?"

"He's hanging in there. We spoke yesterday morning and he acted like everything was fine."

"He acted," Donna repeated, frowning.

Mel shrugged. "I'm supposed to have lunch with him today. Maybe he'll open up and tell me what's really going on."

Donna nodded. "Let me know if there's anything that I can do – for either of you."

"I will."

***

Brad sank into a chair behind the nurse's station and pressed his index fingers to his temples.

"What's wrong?" Miriam asked. "Headache?"

"Something like that," he said.

She watched him for a moment. "So I see we're both off tomorrow. How about we go fishing?" She asked.

"I don't know," he said. "I've got some things I need to take care of tomorrow." He closed his eyes and massaged his temples again.

"Like what?"

"Just… things."

"So some other time then?"

Brad exhaled. "Maybe. Sure."

Miriam watched him for a moment, studying his face. Then she surprised him when she reached out and took his hand into hers, pulling him to his feet.

"Come with me. Let's take a walk," she said.

"To where?"

"You'll see when we get there." She led him to the elevator and they stepped in together. Miriam pressed a button, and it stopped at the fourth floor.

Labor and Delivery.

Brad had walked these halls a few times before, when he and Sue had come to visit friends and family members who had delivered babies.

However, this was the first time that he'd ever set foot on the unit as a nurse, not a visitor. He followed Miriam as they took a right turn and journeyed to the nurse's station at the Labor and Delivery North unit. "Wait here," Miriam instructed Brad, as she ducked behind the desk and tapped the shoulder of a fellow nurse. After a brief conversation, the Labor and Delivery nurse nodded her head, then led Miriam and Brad to another room. She swiped her namebadge through an electronic monitor on the door, which opened with a soft beep.

Miriam and Brad entered a small room full of rocking chairs, sinks, and shelves upon shelves of sterile gowns. Following the Labor and Delivery nurse's lead, Brad and Miriam scrubbed their hands, gloved them, then donned blue hair bonnets and gowns. "Have a seat," the Labor and Delivery nurse directed.

She disappeared behind another closed door, and returned, rolling two bassinets on front of her, each containing a newborn baby.

"Oh," Brad said softly, with realization. Miriam lifted one of the babies and handed it to Brad, and took the other one into her own arms. Instinctively, the nurses held the newborns to their chests, sat down in the rocking chairs, and began to rock them. The Labor and Delivery nurse smiled and left the room, letting them know that she would return in a few minutes to check on the babies.

They rocked and rocked, and caressed the newborns' tiny feet and hands and faces.

"So tiny," Brad murmured dreamily. "And so perfect."

"I know," Miriam responded, with the same sense of awe in her voice. "Babies are beautiful, aren't they?"

"They really are."

They rocked.

"What are their names?" asked Brad.

Miriam looked at the identification cards on the bassinets. "Mine is named Emily Renee. Yours is named Jordan James."

"Hi little Jordan James," Brad whispered. He touched the baby's tiny hand, and grinned with delight as the infant wrapped his miniature fingers around his thumb.

Miriam patted Emily Renee's diapered bottom, and made a face when the tiny girl let out a loud burst of gas. "Peeee-yew," Miriam said, wrinkling her nose. "I haven't smelled gas like that since Homer was alive. This kid could have given him some serious competition."

Both nurses laughed.

They rocked and rocked.

"Miriam?"

"Yes?"

"Not to be blunt but… why are we here? Is this supposed to cheer me up or something? Am I supposed to feel better because these babies have replaced the lives that we lost this week?"

Miriam sighed softly. "No," she replied. "I didn't bring you here thinking that rocking a baby for a few minutes would magically heal your pain. That's not the point."

"I'm not in any pain," Brad said, obviously irritated. "I know I haven't been a nurse for that long, but you all keep forgetting that I was a Navy medic for four years, and a paramedic for another two years. I've seen a lot of people die."

"But I doubt that you ever got attached to them. Not the way you did with Ms. Benson."

"Sure, I liked Ms. Benson. She was sweet. But she's gone. Nothing I can do about that." He shrugged. "It doesn't mean I'm devastated over it."

"You can pretend with the others," Miriam said sternly, "but not with me. I see through it."

"Whatever, Miriam. Just because the rest of you are crying in the break room, acting all touchy-feely, and hugging each other every five minutes doesn't mean that I need the same things. I'm a guy. We deal with things differently than women."

"I know you're a guy," Miriam said. "But you're still human. You still have feelings. You're not that different from us women."

"I'm fine. I swear I am. It's no big deal."

"I remember when I lost my first patient," Miriam continued. "He was a young man, probably about the same age as Devin. He was a construction worker and had fallen from the top of a tall building. Massive TBI. The poor guy never stood a chance." She looked up and away, as if images of the tragic event were being projected from her memory onto the wall.

"That's sad," Brad responded.

"Yes, it was," Miriam echoed. "His name was Donald. Most men named Donald will shorten it to Don, but not him. His nickname was Aldie. He had a young wife and three small children, and death came very unexpectedly for him, just the way it did for Devin. Believe it or not, Brad, I was about your age. And it caught me totally off guard, just like it did for you." She paused as Emily Renee burped. "I'm not sure, but I think Homer may have reincarnated into this baby."

Brad laughed loudly. "This one's pretty quiet. Want to trade?"

"Nope. Keep holding him."

"Okay. But my arm is getting tired." As gently as Brad could, he shifted the baby to rest on his other arm. "Ow," he said loudly when he finished the maneuver. "This little guy is only seven pounds and ten ounces, but if you hold him for long enough, he feels like a bag of bricks. My shoulder is aching like I pinched a nerve or something!"

"I'm sure it is."

"And I only held him for what... like five minutes?"

"Even less," Miriam chided him. "Didn't think it would hurt to hold a baby, did you?'

"Of course not. Why would it?"

"Aha," Miriam said, and turned to Brad. "And that, my dear, is why we're here."

Brad wrinkled his brow in confusion. "Huh?"

"Sometimes you don't realize – or don't want to believe – that something you think is 'no big deal' could be such a heavy burden to bear. And if you don't understand or accept how much it weighs on you, it will catch up with you, all at once, and it will hurt like the devil."

"Miriam," I'm fine, "Brad insisted. "I can't just go around crying over every patient that dies. I'll be emotionally exhausted and I'll never be able to do this job."

"Honey, you'll be emotionally exhausted if you don't."

""I'm not a big fan of crying."

"You don't have to cry. But you need to let it out somehow. You keep it cooped up inside of you and it's going to wear you out so fast, you'll never see it coming."

Miriam stood and put Emily Renee back in her bassinet, and helped Brad do the same for Jordan James. Then they sank back down into their rocking chairs, both of their chests and shoulders burning slightly from baby weight.

"No I don't. I'm fine."

"It's a loss for you too, Brad. Don't trivialize it. Pretending that you're not hurt won't change the way you're feeling inside."

Brad sighed. "So… what makes you so sure that I'm hurting?"

Miriam put her hand on the young nurse's shoulder. "I saw your face when you came back from the ICU, and when you got the call letting you know that Ms. Benson had died. It was a hard moment in your life, and one you'll never forget. And I recognized it because I had a moment just like that, back when my first patient died. I had just left his room and was writing out his vitals on his chart, and then I heard all of this commotion, and saw a frenzy of people rush into his room. And moments later, they came out, and I heard somebody say "Aldie's passed." I just remember thinking about how stupid the whole thing was, because Aldie sounded like "Oldie" when that person said it. Which was kind of ironic because the patient was so young… my God, he was young, and had so much life left in him…just like Devin…" Miriam began to weep.

Brad reached out and touched her arm. "I didn't want Amena to die," he said. "And I didn't want Devin to die either. It just seems so unfair. Both of them on the same day. I couldn't believe it. I thought it was crazy that we live in the twenty-first century and we've got all of the miracles of modern medicine… drugs and surgeries and procedures and therapies… and really, was there nothing, NOTHING at all that we could do to save them? I just couldn't believe it, Miriam, and I still can't."

"I know. It's hard for me, too. But that's just how things are. That's life. Death is part of the package. Look at my Homer. He lived a long and happy life, and his death was expected. We were both prepared for it, had all of the arrangements made, and I lived my life knowing that every day with him could be the last. But that didn't make it any easier when the time came."

Brad watched her cry. "I always wondered how you felt about losing Homer," he said. "You're always joking around about him. You don't seem all that sad."

Miriam shrugged. "I put up a strong front," she said. "If I can laugh and joke about losing him, and convince other people that I'm not hurting, then maybe one of these days, I can convince myself too. But it does hurt, Brad. I do miss him. And I do think about him all the time. I just try not to talk about it."

"It sounds like you need to take your own advice and start letting some of that out."

Nodding, Miriam smiled. "And I guess I am. Right now, with you. I haven't really talked to anyone very much about Homer since he passed." She sniffled.

"I'm sorry about Homer, Miriam."

"I loved him so much, Brad… you have no idea…"

He nodded. "I'm sorry," he said again.

"And I'm sorry about Ms. Benson." Then she added quietly, "And I'm sorry about Sue."

He looked at her and frowned. "No reason to be. Sue didn't die. She just left."

"Still, Brad, so much loss all at once. It hurts. I know it does."

He shook his head. "I'm fine."

Blotting her eyes, Miriam folded her hands over Brad's. "There you go. Denial. The first sign that you're grieving."

Brad laughed and sniffled.

"Do you remember what Aldie looked like before he died?" he continued, quietly. "The last time I saw Amena alive, I knew that death was coming. Her face was so white, like a ghost. And her mouth was wide open, and her head was thrown all the way back... she was having such a hard time breathing, even with oxygen... and I was so sad for her. I just wanted to lay down next to her and hold her, and tell her that everything was going to be alright. It's exactly the way that my Grandma Lillian looked the last time I saw her alive..."

And without warning, he burst into tears. Miriam stood up, took Brad's hands into her own and pulled him to his feet, giving him a strong embrace.

The two nurses held each other tightly and wept until a calm came over them. They let go of each other, blotted their eyes, and looked down at the babies in the bassinets. Both were wriggling furiously.

"I guess little Emily and Jordan think we're saps," Miriam said.

"Probably so," Brad agreed.

"Your shoulder still hurt?"

"A little. Not so much now."

Miriam was nodding. "Good," she said. "That's good. And I have to admit, you were on to me a while ago. There is another reason why I wanted you to spend some time here today."

"Yeah?" Brad looked at her curiously.

"I know you've seen a lot of death and I know you've been able to navigate through it well enough to stay in the game. And I respect that. I know you'll get through this tough time just as well. And this definitely won't be the last time you'll have to deal with a patient dying. You work at a hospital, and that's going to happen, Brad. This place is like a revolving door for life. It comes and goes every day, several times a day, and you're going to see a lot of people die as a nurse."

Miriam reached down and touched wiggling Emily, who made a weird face, passed gas again, and then, very peacefully went to sleep.

"But I wanted you to see the other side of the equation," Miriam said. "I wanted you to see the beginning of life, to be able to touch it and feel it and smell it, and for you to know that you're a part of that too. Life is a journey, and to be there at the beginning or the end of someone else's journey is a privilege. We're not gods, Brad, we're nurses. We don't give life, and we don't save lives or take lives. We're just the ones who make it easier for the person who's coming or going, and we're the ones who support the family and the friends through it. And it can be really, really hard to deal with day in and day out. But..." Miriam reached up to his face and wiped a tear from under his eye with her thumb. "There's a lot of joy that can be found under the roof of Dogwood Regional Medical Center, and you have every right to share in that too."

He smiled.

"There are beautiful new babies, and sick people that get well, and friendships with other nurses, and crazy old women who blow fifteen thousand dollars at bachelor auctions to save their friends from foaming-at-the-mouth doctor's wives. If that's not joy, my friend, I don't know what is."

Brad laughed and took Miriam into his arms again. "I love you, Miriam."

"I love you too, Fishpants. And I'll quit bugging you and let you grieve in whatever way you have to. But keep in mind that I'm here for you, and if there's anything that I can do for you, just ask."

"I know," he said, and glanced at his watch. "Speaking of, I'm going to ask you to let me take off right now, if you don't mind. I need to clock out and head to Amena's funeral. They're doing a short service at the cemetery."

"Go ahead."

He smiled. "If I didn't thank you enough for the fifteen thousand dollar-save, thank you."

"Oh, I know you're thankful," she said with a wink. Then her eyes brightened. "Oh, speaking of that... you know, we won a weekend stay at the beach for bringing in the highest bid. What do you say we all go? Me, you, Haylie, Donna and Mel and their families?"

"I think it's a great idea. Let's do it."

***

Mel knocked on the door of David's office.

"Come in," he said with a smile as he pulled the door open. "How are you doing?"

"I've seen better days," she said. "I guess my spiritual, emotional and mental personal protective equipment has failed me miserably." Mel took a seat.

"Why do you say that?"

Tears sprang to her eyes. "I fell in love with my patient, and then he died on me. I don't know how to dig myself out from underneath all of the feelings and thoughts and the dreams and everything else. I've prayed, I've talked to friends, I'm crying and letting things out, not bottling them up and holding them in... what else can I do?"

"All the above," David said with a quick nod. "Again and again and again. You're doing everything right, Mel. Just keep doing it. Healing is a process, not an event. Right now it probably feels like you're never going to get over this, but you will. It's going to take time."

"I was just told to 'get over it' today by another nurse. She said that since I only knew Devin for a week, I don't have any real right to mourn his loss. Her advice is completely opposite from yours. So who am I supposed to listen to?"

"Yourself," he said. "Your heart and mind and body are telling you what you need to do. When you feel the need to talk about it, you do it. When you feel the need to cry and scream, then do it. There's no such thing as 'just get over it' when it comes to this. You lost a loved one. It doesn't matter if you knew him for a week or a lifetime. You loved him, and now you're having to let go of him, and you're the only one who understands what that feels like."

"But there's the problem... I don't know how to let go," Mel said. "Every time I fall asleep, I dream about him. And in those dreams, he's still alive. And I wake up feeling happy, and as soon as I realize that I was only dreaming, I get really depressed."

David handed her a box of tissues. "So the dreams make you happy?"

"Sure they do. Until I wake up."

Grinning, David crossed his legs and leaned back in his chair. He cupped his chin in his hand thoughtfully. "Why do you say your dreams aren't real?"

Mel looked insulted. "Because he's dead, and all the dreams in the world aren't going to bring him back."

"But they're real to you. While you're dreaming, they make you happy. You feel like Devin's still with you."

"But he's not," Mel cried. "I don't want to pretend. I don't want to wake up. It's like someone is playing a cruel joke on me."

"Maybe you can change the way that you feel about your dreams."

"How?"

"Perhaps your dreams are serving a purpose. Maybe this is your mind's way of helping you to accept reality. Maybe it's too painful for Devin to be taken away from you right now, so you're only having to let go of him when you're awake."

"I don't know," Mel shrugged. "It's wonderful until I wake up."

David paused for a moment. "Where do you think Devin is now, Mel?"

"Heaven... I think. I hope."

"So you believe that Devin has a soul and that it's still alive, and in Heaven."

"I want to believe that, anyway."

"Maybe that's where he is, then. Maybe your dreams are real, and you can really see Devin spiritually, just not physically."

Mel sighed. "Now you sound like Devin's mother. She told me about the night that Devin was born, she and her husband were in a car accident. The accident killed her husband, but she said that she remembers him being there with her in the hospital when Devin was born. Like his soul detached from his body and stayed with her until their son was born. And I have no doubt that she believes it really happened, but I just don't believe in that kind of stuff. I'm Catholic. I believe that when people die, people go to an afterlife, and they don't come back. I don't believe in ghosts and lingering spirits."

"I'm surprised to hear that," David said. "Because being Catholic shouldn't put you at odds with believing in things of that nature."

Mel's eyebrows shot up as David reached for a Bible on his desk. He opened it to the book of Mark, and pointed to Chapter 9, beginning with verse 2. "Read the next couple of verses," he said.

Mel read them aloud:

"And after six days Jesus taketh with him Peter, and James, and John, and leadeth them up into a high mountain apart by themselves: and he was transfigured before them. And his raiment became shining, exceeding white as snow; so as no fuller on earth can white them. And there appeared unto them Elijah with Moses: and they were talking with Jesus."

Mel paused.

"Do you know who Elijah and Moses are?"

"Of course I do," she said. "From the Old Testament. They were long gone before Jesus, Peter, James and John came into the picture."

"Right. They were dead."

Mel looked up at David. "So Elijah and Moses were…"

"Apparitions, ghosts, spirits…those are some of the words that have been used to describe this story from the Bible."

"And it wasn't just Jesus who saw them. Peter, James, and John witnessed it. They saw the… apparitions… too."

David nodded. "What do you think, after reading that?"

Mel shrugged and closed the Bible, handing it back to David. "I'm not sure," she said.

"Seeing is believing," he said. "Jesus saw Elijah and Moses, and so did the three disciples. Did that make them real?"

"Maybe. I don't know," Mel said.

"And that's okay," David said with a smile. "You don't have to have all the answers, Mel. There are some things we'll never understand. Especially as health care professionals – we live and breathe science every single day, and we're very uncomfortable with things that we can't measure. We tend to think that things that can't be measured aren't real."

Mel crossed her arms, deep in thought. "Like pain," she said. "None of us really knew how to deal with pain until we put numbers on it to quantify it."

"Exactly. But if you don't put a number on pain, does that mean it doesn't exist?"

"Of course not, she said. I see patients in horrible pain. There's no question in my mind it's real."

"And there are other things that are hard to quantify. Like love," David said. "People tried to tell you that you couldn't possibly be in love with Devin."

"But I was," she said, wiping a tear from her cheek. "And I still am."

"That love remains very real to you."

"Of course it does."

"So thinking about things like love and pain... perhaps it's not such a stretch to think that there are other things in life that can be real, without being able to be measured."

"Maybe," Mel said quietly.

"You're not that different from others, Mel. Most widows experience the presence of their deceased husbands within a year after the loss. And most parents who have lost a child experience the presence of that child within a year after the loss."

"In dreams?"

"Quite often, yes. And some claim to see apparitions. Some claim to hear voices or smell a fragrance associated with their lost loved one. Others just feel a presence."

"Could that many people just be imagining things?"

David shrugged. "I couldn't even begin to speculate on how or why those experiences happen for the loved ones left behind. All I'm telling you, Mel, is that you and Beverly are not that different from others. Most people who lose a very close loved one have a personal experience in which they sense the presence of that loved one after their death. So you're in good company."

She sat quietly for a moment. "I think I get it," she said softly, more to herself than to David. "It's all personal and individual."

"Pardon me?" He asked, cupping his hand to his ear to let her know that he hadn't been able to hear her comment.

"Sorry," she apologized. "I'm just thinking out loud here. About the difference between believing and knowing," she said. "I had a conversation with Devin's mother. We talked about how there are some things that we believe because we have faith but we can't prove them. And then there are some things that we know, because we have proof – even if the proof belongs to us alone. I guess Jesus, Peter, James and John didn't have any room for doubt when they saw Elijah and Moses with their own eyes. They knew it was real."

They sat quietly for a moment.

"It sounds as though your mind might be a little more open now than when you first walked in," David said.

"It is," she said, exhaling deeply. "Once again, you've helped me more than you'll ever know." She stood to return to work.

"More than I'll ever know?" He asked with a smile. "Then I'll just believe." He rose from his chair to see her to the door. "Can we share a word of prayer before you leave, Mel?"

"Please," she said, bowing her head and wiping tears from her eyes. "I need all of the help I can get."

He laid a caring hand on her shoulder, and together they prayed.

***

Amena Benson's yard was so full of cars that Brad had to parallel park in a tiny space on the cul-de-sac. Inside the house, there were even more people, making it an even tighter squeeze.

The room buzzed like a beehive with the chatter of visitors who came to pay their respects to Ms. Benson's family. Brad recognized several faces in the crowd. Several of them were Amena's fellow volunteers and employees from Dogwood Regional. Glancing around, he saw Cassandra lingering in a doorway and staring down at her tiny plate of cocktail sausages, cheese cubes and crackers. Brad pushed his way toward her, and she looked up as he approached.

"Hi," she said, her face brightened. "If you'd like to get something to eat, there's plenty of food in the kitchen."

Brad shook his head. "Thanks, but I'm not really hungry."

"Neither am I," Cassandra said, looking down at her plate with disgust. "They just buried my mother. Food is the last thing on my mind. Isn't it crazy that this is what people do after funerals? They get together… and eat?"

Smiling, Brad looked at her sympathetically. "It does seem kind of stupid," he says. "The eating part, I mean. Maybe food is just our excuse to get together one more time before we have to say goodbye."

Just then, a heavyset elderly woman approached and stood between Brad and Cassandra, gently touching her on the arm. "Darling, I'm so sorry about your mother. If you need anything, please call me, won't you?"

"Yes Ma'am, I certainly will." Cassandra forced a smile as the woman shuffled away, then turned her attention back to Brad. "It's weird, you know. With all of these people here, it kind of feels like she's still here."

"How so?"

"Well, everyone here was part of her life. I haven't seen all my family together under one roof since Christmas. This is where we've always met for Christmas, at Mom's house. For as long as I can remember. The minute you walked in the door, you could smell hot apple cider and turkey in the oven, you could feel the warmth from the fireplace. And of course, Mom would make stockings for all of the grandkids, and every year they'd be hanging there with an early present from Santa. Santa, being my mother, of course. She would always be running back and forth between the kitchen and the living room, not wanting to miss a minute of anything. And I can still see her, standing right here, right where I am now."

"The way you describe it, I can almost see her too," Brad said.

Cassandra smiled. "And those ladies over there – you see the two sitting on the piano bench, and the third one standing up and talking to them?" She pointed at the group she was referring to.

"Yes. Are they family?"

"They're not relatives, but they're about as close as you can get to family. They're her lifelong friends Ginger, Dot, and Carol. Believe it or not, they were all born and raised here in Dogwood, were neighbors on the same street and went to school together all the way through high school. They've always been close. We called them the 'Fabulous Four.' You never saw just two or three of them together – always the four of them. They were a set."

"So I guess it looks pretty strange to see the three of them now …"

"No," she said, shaking her head. "That's the weirdest thing. When I look at the three of them, it's like Mom's still there. She wouldn't dream of letting those three get together without her, so I figure she can't be too far away."

Brad braced himself, feeling certain that another monologue about the glorious afterlife and Amena's spirit dancing on clouds was coming. *Please… no more heaven and eternity and religion talk. I got my fill of it at the funeral.*

Cassandra sighed and looked down at her plate again. "I'm not going to eat this food, do you want it?"

Brad was relieved that she had changed the subject. "No thanks," he replied.

"Well let's go give it to Bella."

"Who's Bella?"

"Come with me," she said, taking him by the elbow and weaving through the crowd into the kitchen, then through a sliding glass door to the back yard. "Bella! Bell-Bell, come here, honey!" She called.

A droopy-eyed basset hound poked her head out of a doghouse nestled in the far corner of the fenced yard. "Aroooo!" She hollered back to Cassandra.

"Bella, come here! Food!" She put the plate down in front of her feet, and Brad watched as the long-bodied dog with stubby legs emerged from its shelter and galloped across the yard, her ears twirling around like pinwheels and drool flying from her mouth.

Brad couldn't help but laugh. "She's cute," he said, kneeling down to her as she gobbled up Cassandra's food.

"Go for it, girl," Cassandra said. "A last meal for you."

Brad's smile faded. "Last meal? What?"

"Well, sadly, I'm going to have to take her to the shelter later today."

Brad looked up at her. "You're getting rid of her?" He asked.

"She was my Mom's dog," she explained. "Now that Mom's not here anymore, I don't know what to do with her. I can't take her because I'm allergic to pet dander. And I can't talk anyone in my family into taking her home."

"Where are you taking her?"

"Dogwood County Animal Control," she said.

The words sent a chill up Brad's spine. "But you know what they'll do if she doesn't get adopted, don't you?"

"Yes. They'll put her to sleep in three days. I already called and they told me their policies."

"Three days? Are you serious?"

"Their shelter's full. It's unfortunate, but they don't have a choice."

"Well… wait a minute… you know Miriam from my unit? She volunteers at the Humane Society. I don't think they euthanize. I bet if we talk to Miriam, she could work something out—"

"Already did," Cassandra said, sadly. "Miriam told me that if she could pull strings and get Bella in, she would. But it's not up to her. The shelter managers have to make some tough decisions, and right now they can't take any more animals in because they don't have the resources to care for them."

Brad reached out and let the dog sniff him, as Miriam had taught him to do. She wagged her tail and licked his palm. Then he stroked the side of her face with his finger tips. "She's a nice dog." He looked into her droopy eyes, and his heart melted.

"She sure is. I hate to do this. But I've asked everyone that I know." Cassandra began to cry. "This wasn't supposed to happen, you know. Mom was the big dog lover in the family. She was supposed to outlive the dog, not the other way around. And now that she's not here… I don't want to do this, Brad. I don't want to have to visit my mother's grave and let her know that I couldn't find a home for Bella. She loved her so much."

Brad stood up and touched Cassandra's shoulder.

And he prayed.

May there be peace in the world far and near, and may I bring peace to the person right here.

"You didn't ask everybody," he said.

She looked confused. "You?" She asked. "You would take her in?"

"Hey, you said I did a wonderful job taking care of your mother... wouldn't you trust me with her dog?" He smiled. "I'd be honored if I could give Bella a home."

"You mean it? You could really do this?"

He nodded. "I loved your mother too, Cassandra. I think if I adopt Bella, it will help keep her close to me."

Cassandra threw her arms around Brad, nearly knocking him over. "Thank you.... Oh, thank you, Brad. I don't know how to thank you."

Bella licked the last few bits of food from the paper plate. She looked up at Brad and Cassandra, belched and wagged her tail.

"That's my kind of dog," Brad said. "We're going to get along just fine."

"Thank you," Cassandra said again, wiping tears from her eyes.

Brad was touched by her concern for the dog, and thought he saw a new side of Cassandra Putnam that was reasonably selfless; almost sweet and almost endearing.

"You know, Brad, if you want, I can come by your place on occasion to check on her, and see how you two are doing," she offered, and shot Brad a flirtatious look.

Almost endearing, Brad thought to himself. *But not quite.*

"I think we'll be okay," he said, forcing a smile.

Chapter 15
Wednesday

"Really, Donna... aren't the disguises just a wee bit over the top?" Miriam fidgeted with the baseball cap on her head and grumbled. "I thought that was why I'm driving my truck. If no one recognizes the vehicle, they're not going to pay attention to the passengers." She drummed her fingers on the steering wheel.

"I'm not taking any chances," Donna said, cowering below the dashboard as she adjusted a pair of dark sunglasses over her eyes and tucked a stray strand of hair back into the scarf she had tied around her forehead.

"Explain to me again what we're doing?" Miriam said impatiently.

"We're stalking my son," she replied.

"And why, exactly?"

Donna sighed. "Since he's been out of prison, he's been acting like the perfect angel."

Miriam looked at her out of the corner of her eye. "And that's a problem?"

"I need to know if it's sincere," Donna said. "I want to believe, but the skeptic in me doesn't think that a leopard can change its spots all that easily."

"The skeptic in you never did hard time behind bars, either.

Maybe Darius really has changed. What reason do you have to doubt him?"

"I don't. But there's a sneakiness about him. Phone calls early in the morning and late at night. And making plans to meet up with old friends. His 'dawgs,' as he puts it," Donna said with disgust.

"Hmmm," Miriam murmured. "That sounds downright scandalous, Donna. How do you sleep at night? With one eye open, I hope."

Donna swatted Miriam on the arm playfully. "Quit mocking me."

"Quit hitting me. That was an assault. Who's the criminal now, eh Donna?"

"Miriam!" She growled. "I need for you to take this seriously." She jolted up in her seat. "There he is," she said, pointing at her son emerging from a cell phone store on foot. "Start the engine. Follow him. Not too close, we don't want him to figure out we're on his trail."

Miriam turned the key and the truck purred to life. "Which one of Charlie's Angels are you, anyway?"

A tall man stepped out of the cell phone store behind Darius, wearing blue jeans that drooped in the back so that his boxer shorts were showing.

"Ooooooh!" Donna nearly screamed. "I'd like to jump out of this truck and go pull his pants up. Shame on him!" She pointed at Darius' friend. "You see that? That's the kind of rubbish that got my son into trouble in the first place."

Miriam shook her head. "I see what you mean. Just where are the fashion police when you need them? Can't trust a man if you can see his underwear, that's what I always say."

"Would you quit picking on me?" Donna asked.

"No. Are you kidding me? That's in style right now. I see young men dressed like that all the time. It doesn't mean anything. Get a grip, Donna."

"Follow that car," she commanded, as Darius and the friend with the boxers climbed into a black, older model sedan and pulled out of the parking lot. Miriam pulled out into traffic and followed at a distance.

"I bet Darius just bought a prepaid cell phone," Donna fumed.

Miriam pretended to shriek. "I've got a prepaid cell phone too, Donna. Are you going to turn me into the police?"

"You don't understand," Donna said. "A prepaid cell phone is a dealer's best friend. You use it to do all of your dirty business and the calls can't be traced."

"I think you're overreacting."

They followed the sedan for another few miles, until it took a turn into a shady looking neighborhood.

"I don't like the looks of this," Donna said.

"Then close your eyes."

"Just drive, Miriam." Donna sighed.

The sedan took another turn, onto a winding service road with no street sign posted. It pulled into a parking lot and parked behind a rickety looking building. Several other cars were parked in the lot, and a crowd of young men around Darius' age stood together in a circle, talking. Each of them had a small, square object in their hands. Darius and his friend, each with a similar object in their hands, left the sedan and joined the circle.

"Oh my God," Donna whispered. "Where are we? A crackhouse? And who are all of those men? And what are they holding? Boxes of some kind? It has to be drugs, Miriam. DRUGS. Oh my Lord. Or guns."

Miriam shook her head. "You're jumping to conclusions. Just relax."

"I will not relax," Donna snapped, "and I will not harbor a criminal that lies to my face about being a changed man and a good Christian," she said, the pitch of her voice rising with each word until she was nearly screaming. She unbuckled her seat belt and threw the truck door open.

"What are you doing?" Miriam asked, obviously shocked.

"I'm going to give my son a piece of my mind," she said. She stomped across the parking lot, pulling the scarf off of her head and tossing the sunglasses onto the pavement.

"Darius Phillip LeShay!" She blurted out.

Upon hearing his name, Darius turned away from his conversation with his friend. He did a double-take as he saw Donna approaching.

"Mama?" He said, obviously confused.

"That's right it's your Mama!" She screamed. "I'd like to know what exactly it is you think you're doing here, and who all these thugs are! And don't you lie to me! I brought you into this world, and I will TAKE YOU OUT OF IT if you tell me one more lie!"

All eyes were on Donna as she went into meltdown mode. A couple of the men took a step back, distancing themselves from Darius.

"Mama," he said calmly, "I haven't lied to you."

"You told me you changed! That you'd given your life to the Lord!"

"I did," he said.

"So what business do you have with these people?"

Darius pointed to a sign in the corner of the parking lot, just on the other side of the run-down building. A single piece of plywood was mounted in the ground on a stake, and the words "Urban Ministries" were painted on it, with a cross and the sign of the fish underneath.

Donna felt her stomach flop.

"I'm here for Bible study, Mama," Darius said.

She looked at the rectangular-shaped objects in the men's hands. They were Bibles.

"I was invited here to give my testimony," Darius continued. "There are lots of young men in this community that have had run-ins with the law, and I wanted to tell them what life in prison is like and how they can make different choices. I'm going to tell my story and share with them how choosing to follow God's Will saved my life."

Donna could feel her heart breaking. Never in her life had she felt so ashamed of herself.

"Oh son," she said, as tears begin to spill from her eyes. "I'm... I'm sorry. You just had me worried, you know, all those late night and early morning phone calls. Speaking of... what were you doing at the cell phone store?"

"I went to meet Joe," Darius said, pointing to his friend. "He works there. And at an auto shop. And as a server in a restaurant a couple of days a week. It's hard to find time to stay in touch with him, because no matter what time of day it is, he's always at work. That's why I usually talk to him really late at night or really early in the morning."

Like a perfect gentleman, Joe extended his hand and shook Donna's. "Pleased to meet you," he said.

Darius continued. "Joe and I were tangled up in the same mess together, and ended up in prison about the same time. But we decided to clean up our acts, and help others through some hard times."

Donna's jaw dropped to the ground. "Okay... but what about Fang? Who's Fang?"

Darius and Joe laughed. "Come with me, Mama," Darius said, taking her by the hand and leading her to the sedan. The window on the driver's side was rolled down, and Darius poked his head through. "Fang," he said. "Come say hello to my mom."

Donna peered into the car and saw a tiny mixed-breed dog – a graying terrier or chihuahua mix of some kind – shivering on the armrest. He appeared thoroughly uninterested in making her acquaintance. "Uhff," he barked.

"Fang's fourteen years old," Joe explained. "I guess the name isn't all that fitting now that he's lost most of his teeth, but trust me, he was a beast back in the day."

Darius laughed. "Joe got out eight months before me, and he and Fang would come visit me on the weekends sometimes while I was still in."

"He's a dog," Donna said softly to herself. "Not a dawg."

"Are you okay, Mama?" Darius asked.

She faced him, shaking her head. "I'm so sorry, Honey. I know I probably embarrassed the living daylights out of you, but I just had to know the truth."

He wrapped his arms around her. "It's okay. I'm not upset. I put you through hell back then, Mama. You have every right to doubt me."

"Yes I do," she said. "But I don't want to, son. I want to believe in you. I dreamed about having you back in my life for so long, and now that it's finally happened, it caught me off guard. I didn't realize that it would require some getting used to."

"And learning to trust me again," he said. "I understand. Take as long as you need."

She squeezed him. "I'm glad you feel that way. Because I can't promise I'm going to quit being nosy any time soon."

"And that's okay," he said with a smile. "Hey, how did you get here anyway? I don't see your car."

"Miriam and I followed you." She pointed at the truck. Miriam honked the horn and waved. "She's part of my other family. We take care of each other."

Darius smiled. "Do you want to come in? We're going to start Bible study in about fifteen minutes. You both are welcome."

"No," Donna shook her head. "Go ahead, son. I'll see you when you get home. When will you be there?"

"I'm not sure," he said. "But I'll call you and let you know if it's going to be late." He leaned forward and surprised her by taking her into his arms for a hug. "Just trust me, Mama."

"I trust you," she whispered in his ear. "But I love you a whole lot more."

***

When she reached the stairwell to her apartment, she cursed herself for not remembering to leave the porch light on.

A dark figure moved in front of her door, and Mel jumped back. "Bruce!" She screamed. "I told you to never come back here!"

"Hey, it's just me," a soothing male voice said. The voice was familiar, but it wasn't Bruce's. "I didn't mean to scare you." He stepped away from the porch and down the steps and into the light from the street lamps.

Rodney.

He had a vase filled with flowers in his arms. "I've been meaning to call and check on you, to see if you got your car fixed. Is everything okay?"

Mel sighed. "Oh, yeah. It was the timing belt. I got it fixed. Thanks again for giving me a ride back home the other day."

"It was my pleasure," Rodney smiled. Then he looked down at

the vase in his hands. "Oh, the reason I'm here…" he stepped forward and gave it to Mel. " I just wanted to let you know that I was thinking about you. I hope you don't mind, but I was just going to leave some flowers on your doorstep."

Mel looked down at the flowers in her arms. "It's so dark, I can't tell what they are," she said.

"They're sunflowers."

She smiled. "Thank you," she said. "With the twelve-hour shifts I work, I don't get to see the sunshine very often. "

"You told me that on our date," Rodney said. "I thought maybe these would make your day just a little bit brighter." He handed the bouquet to her. "I hope you'll call me sometime if you'd like to get together again, Mel. Take care."

He kissed her cheek, then stepped past her, making his way to leave.

"Rodney?" she called out.

He turned. "Yes?"

Don't go, she wanted to say.

But instead, she steeled herself. "Thank you."

Halfway up the stairs to her apartment, her mobile phone rang. Wedging the vase in the crook of her arm, she fumbled inside of her handbag.

"Hello?" She asked, after pressing the phone to her ear.

"Hi," Bruce said. "How are you doing?"

"I've had better days," she replied.

"I've been thinking about you."

"Uh huh," Mel said, absentmindedly. She reached the top of the stairwell and stopped at the door.

"How's Jenny?"

"She's fine, other than an occasional bout of morning sickness."

Bruce sighed. "Poor Jen. I remember how rough it was for you when you were pregnant with her. You were sick every single morning, remember?"

"How could I forget?" Mel said, and laughed softly.

Bruce hesitated for a moment. "Mel, have you thought any more about what I said the other day?"

"Yes," she said. "I've actually thought about it a lot."

"And?"

"And I need to tell you something."

"Okay," Bruce said expectantly.

Mel took a deep breath. "I forgive you," she said.

"Mel," Bruce said, his voice strained with emotion, "does this mean—"

"No," she quickly said. "We're not getting back together, Bruce. I'm sorry, but too much damage has been done to our marriage for me to ever trust you or love you again. But I recognize that you regret the things that happened, and I believe you when you say that you're sorry. So I forgive you."

Bruce was silent on the other end of the line.

"I forgive you," Mel repeated. "For the sake of our children, and our grandchild. And for me. Life is too short to carry around so much anger, so I'm letting it all go."

"I am sorry," Bruce said. He began to cry. "I'm just so sorry, Mel, for everything I did to screw up our marriage. You do deserve better, and I hope... I pray that you will find someone who makes you happy. Who loves you the way you deserve to be loved."

Mel looked at the sunflowers spilling out of the vase in her arms and smiled. "Thank you," she said. "I know you're sorry, but that's all in the past. Let's consider this a new beginning."

"Beginning of what?"

"Peace between you and me," Mel said. "I know it may not be everything that you want, but—"

"It's enough," Bruce said. "Thank you, Mel."

Chapter 16
Thursday

Joann was surprised to find Haylie's car in the driveway. Her daughter hadn't come to visit since she had moved out a few weeks ago, and Joann suspected Haylie was trying to make the point that she was doing just fine on her own.

Haylie hadn't called her mother very much and had been slow to return her calls.

Joann suspected that it was just a phase. Just a newly independent young woman proving to herself, and to her mother, that she really was going to be okay on her own. Once Haylie got herself altogether, Joann was sure that they would be close again.

"Haylie?" Joann called out, as she stepped inside the house.

She remembered how Haylie had tried her best to take the house key off of her keyring and give it back to Joann the day she moved out.

"I want you to keep it," Joann had told her.

"Mom! I have my own home now."

"I know. But this will always be your home too. You're a lucky person, Haylie. You have two homes."

"I don't need two homes. If I want to come over and visit, I'll just knock and you can let me in. I don't need a key."

"Yes you do. I live alone now. What if there's an emergency? You're my next of kin. I may need for you to be able to get into the house at some point. Please, Haylie, keep the key."

Reluctantly, she had kept it. Joann was glad that she had insisted. "Haylie?" she called again, as she walked down the hallway toward her daughter's old room.

Joann found her daughter curled up on top of her old twin bed. Haylie's entire body was wrapped, full fetal position, around her old pillow. "Honey, what's wrong?" Joann asked, as she approached the bed and sat down next to her.

Haylie looked up. Her eyes were bloodshot and her cheeks were wet.

Joann instinctively reached out and pressed the palm of her hand to Haylie's forehead. "Are you sick, honey? What's wrong?"

"I looked all over the store," Haylie said, her voice trembling. "I looked all over the store, and I still couldn't find the right detergent. I know it's in a bottle that looks pink or purple and has bees on it, and the bottle says something like 'smells sweet as honey'… or something like that, but I still couldn't find the right one."

Joann looked confused. "What?"

"I went to three different stores, Mom. I opened all the bottles and sniffed them, and I still couldn't find the one that you use." Her eyes shimmered as new tears formed. "If I can't find the right detergent, then how in the world am I ever going to make it on my own?"

Joann laughed softly and put her arms around Haylie, pulling her up to a sitting position as she hugged her. "Honey, there is no right detergent. You can choose whichever one you want. And it's okay if you pick something different from what I use. That's why there are so many brands, honey. Because different people like different things. There's no right or wrong when it comes to washing clothes."

Haylie wiped her eyes. "I tried washing my laundry with other brands. None of them smell right. None of them smell like home."

Hugging her tighter, Joann laughed again. "Honey, you could have called me. I haven't gone anywhere. I'm right here. Just because you have your own place to live doesn't mean I'm not your mother anymore."

"I know," Haylie said. "I just wish I had figured it out sooner."

"I missed you so much," Joann said.

"I missed you too," Haylie admitted. "And my pillowcase at my place stinks like cheap detergent. What's the right kind, Mom?" Tears spilled down her cheeks.

Joann laughed. "It's called Bee Soft."

"Bee Soft," Haylie repeated. "How in the world could I have forgotten a name like that?" She laughed.

"I think I've got an extra bottle of it in the laundry room," Joann said. "You're welcome to take it home."

Okay," she said. Her face brightened, but only for a second. Suddenly, she was crying all over again.

Joann took her daughter's hands into her own. "This isn't about laundry detergent, is it, honey? What's wrong? Are you just homesick?"

Haylie shook her head. "No," she said. "I really love living by myself in my new apartment, but it can get lonely sometimes. I've had a tough week at work, and when I came home today and felt like the walls were closing in on me, I finally realized that I just needed to talk to a friend. So I came to see my *best* friend."

Joann smiled. "I'm all yours, sweetheart. Talk to me."

Haylie turned to face her mother. She squeezed her hands, and gave a brave smile as tears continued to spill down her face. Then she took a deep breath.

"I lost my first patients this week," she said. "Not just one, but two of them…"

Chapter 17
Friday Evening

Donna's mini-van had never been so jam-packed. Darius had accepted the navigator role and was riding shotgun with directions and a state map resting on his lap. Jeanette and Haylie were sitting in the bench seat in the back of the van, poring through a gossip magazine's special tribute edition to Devin Ryan. Mel, Jenny and Michael piled into the middle seat.

"Michael – get that seat belt on. You too, Jenny. Buckle up that grandbaby of mine," Mel ordered her daughter.

"We're way ahead of you, Mom," Jenny replied, as she and her brother fastened their seat belts.

"So my mom's reputation as a bad driver precedes her," Darius laughed over his shoulder.

"Oh, no… it's nothing like that," Mel said. "I'm just a fan of playing it safe."

Donna glared at her son. "Better quit picking on me, or I'll drop you off at Joe's house and you can spend the weekend sleeping on the couch with that creepy trembling mutt of his."

"Creepy trembling mutt?" Mel asked with a laugh. "I don't even want to know."

"Hey, speaking of mutts," Haylie piped in, "Brad is bringing his dog with him. Have you guys seen her yet? Cute little thing."

"Yes, I heard," Donna said. "That's why he's riding with Miriam and not me."

"Mama's not much of a dog person, in case you couldn't tell," Darius explained with a laugh.

"But you'll love this dog, I bet," Mel said. "I've only seen pictures of her at work on his locker, but I love her already. I think she saved Brad, in a way. She brought him back from the sad place he was in. And oh, what a proud doggie parent he is. He's worse than Miriam is, always showing off pictures of her grandson."

"It sounds like Miriam and Brad have both been blessed," Donna said. "Now they've both got someone new in their lives to love."

"And I'll join the ranks soon when grandbaby Page joins us," Mel said.

"And I got my Darius back," Donna said, touching him on the shoulder.

"Well now I'm feeling left out," Haylie joked. "But then again, I don't think I need any babies or pets in my life to take care of right now."

"Are we there yet?" Michael piped in, as he pulled the earphones out of his ears and joined the conversation.

"We're just getting started, honey," Donna answered in a motherly tone of voice. "It's a long ride to the beach."

***

Three hours later, Donna's mini-van, followed by Miriam's truck, pulled into the gravel parking lot of the beachfront guest house. Miriam pulled the keys out of an envelope and walked up the stairway to the front door. The rest of the nurses and their guests excitedly lined up behind her, one person on every other step, balancing beach chairs and overnight bags. All except for Brad, who was walking Bella on a leash and babytalking her while she sniffed out the perfect spot to relieve herself on a nearby patch of grass.

Inside the house, everyone quickly claimed a bedroom. Except for Brad, who settled in the living room and decided to sleep in the fold-out sofabed as it was the closest accommodations to the sliding glass door, for Bella's benefit.

After everyone settled in and unpacked, they each changed into warm weather clothes and flip flops, and headed to the beachfront. They walked to the shoreline and wet their feet in the cool ocean, talking and laughing.

The sun was just beginning to set when Mel asked the question. "Should we start now?"

Everyone looked at each other and nodded, then retreated onto the sand.

"Let's stand in a circle," Mel suggested.

So they did, and they joined hands and stood in solidarity.

For a long moment, they allowed silence to fill the space between them. The crash of the waves on the shore and the cry of a distant seagull were just barely audible.

And then Mel started.

"Thank you all for agreeing to be a part of this," she said softly.

Jenny, who was standing to her right side, squeezed her hand. Michael squeezed her other hand on the left.

"We're all here – some of us with family," she said, as she cast sideways glances at her own children, and then at Donna, "and some of us, with new friends," she said, winking at Brad, who stood across the circle from her. Bella was resting at his feet. "But we've all come for the same reason. We're here to celebrate the lives of two friends." She paused. "Amena Benson," she said, "And Devin Ryan."

A long silence followed.

The sun began to set in the sky, casting a soft orange glow across the surface of the water.

"This is a time," Mel resumed, "for us to remember our friends, and what they meant to us. This is a time that we can share our thoughts with each other, or keep them to ourselves. This is a time that we can send up prayers and hopes – or just reflect and remember." She smiled and looked around the circle, taking a moment to focus on each face. "If anyone feels led to share, then feel free to start us off."

Brad smiled at her from across the circle. "I'll start," he said with a little laugh. "I want to say goodbye to my friend, Amena Benson."

Everyone focused their attention on him.

He took a deep breath and continued. "Where in the world do I start?" He laughed softly.

Tears began to form in Mel's eyes. Donna's face melted into empathy, and her eyes watered as well.

Brad continued. "Some of you know Amena because she was a volunteer at Dogwood Regional. That's how I met her. Last year, about this time, she came onto the unit with a wheelchair, ready to transport a patient that we were discharging. I remember seeing her for the first time. I remember the way that her big blue eyes and her smile just lit up the room." He looked out at the ocean. "She walked into the patient's room and said, 'Hello darling, your chariot awaits!' And the patient laughed, and sat up in bed. He was a big guy. Close to three hundred pounds. He made some kind of a comment about how Amena was so small, and wondered how in the world she would have the strength to push him out the door. And Amena looked back at him and said, 'have faith in me, dear. If you have faith you can move mountains. So a wheelchair should be no big deal.' And that was my first impression of Amena," Brad said, as his eyes suddenly began to shimmer. "I'll never forget that day."

Tears flowed among the rest of the group

"And since then, every time I would see her coming down the hallway to Med-Surg South, in her cute little pink jacket, and that big smile on her face, I would look at that tiny little woman and say to myself, 'there's a lady who can move mountains.' And just recently…" Brad paused, as he tore his hand away from Donna's long enough to wipe his eyes, "She became the lady who gave me a way to move past something very difficult. Which surprised me more than the thought of her moving a mountain ever could," he said with a smile.

Donna squeezed one of his hands. Haylie squeezed the other.

"I hope that you found peace, Amena," Brad said, a bit more softly. "And if you can hear me or see me, I want you to know that I'll be taking good care of Bella. She'll always have a home with me." He looked down at the basset hound, who had flopped on her side and was resting in the sand. Upon hearing her name, she raised her head up and looked at Brad, then thumped her tail on the sand. "We'll both miss you a lot, Amena," Brad said. "But we'll always remember you."

Another silence fell upon the group, until Donna broke it a few minutes later.

"Rest in peace, Amena," she said. "I trust you have found that glorious peace that Brad wished for you."

Haylie sniffled. "I wish you peace, too, Ms. Benson," she said.

"Thank you for being a friend to all of us," Mel said in a whisper.

"I hope you got to trade in your pink jacket for something really neat, like a pair of wings, Amena," Miriam said.

Everyone laughed. And then they fell into silence again.

"I... I want to say goodbye to Devin," Haylie said. "I guess you all know, he was my big celebrity crush, and never in a million years would I have imagined that he'd end up as a patient on our unit."

Donna laughed. "I thought I was going to have to put a leash on you to keep you out of his room," she said.

"I'm sorry," Haylie grinned. "I couldn't help it."

"Well, he didn't quite have that effect on me," Brad laughed. "But I enjoyed his movies, and I'm glad I got to meet him. I wish he hadn't died so young," Brad said softly. "But I wish him peace also."

"Maybe he's flirting with Amena in heaven right now," Miriam offered. "I never saw his movies, but after meeting him, I have to say - he was quite the charmer. He even made this old woman's heart race a time or two."

The nurses laughed.

"Why is everyone laughing?" Michael whispered to his mother. "I thought this was supposed to be like a funeral or something."

"It's a memorial service, honey. It doesn't have to be sad. We're here to share stories and happy memories, too."

"Oh," Michael said. "So then... can I say something about Devin too?"

"Sure," Mel said. "Speak up so everyone else can hear."

Michael looked shyly at the others around the circle. "I loved all of Devin's movies," he said. "But his last movie was my favorite, because my family saw it together. It's one of the last times that we were all together. My Dad, my Mom, Jenny and I... we went out to celebrate

Mom's birthday for dinner, and then we went to see Devin's movie. And we had a really good time. It was just a really happy day," he said. "Things were kind of... more normal back then, I guess. I just really liked it when we went out together as a family."

Mel blinked and a tear ran down her cheek. She felt ashamed that she had been so focused on herself that she hadn't given much thought to the fact that Jenny and Michael were still grieving a loss of their own.

"I know things can't be the same as before," Michael said, directing his comments to Mel, "but it doesn't mean we have to change everything. Maybe you and me and Jenny could go to the movies sometime – just the three of us? You know, start our own tradition. That could be fun."

"And maybe we can celebrate your birthday this year, Mom?" Jenny asked.

Mel gave a shadow of a smile, but didn't comment.

"I bet Devin would have done something huge for you, Mom," Jenny said. "Had he known your birthday was coming up, he probably would have sent you a bouquet of flowers that would have been ten times as big as the chicken man's bouquet."

More laughter.

"Hey," Mel said, playfully defensive, "I kind of like the chicken man. And his name is Rodney, if you'll recall, and you're the one who picked him out for me, by the way."

"Just kidding," Jenny said with a wink.

A short silence passed.

"Mel?" Donna prompted her. "You were the closest to Devin of all of us," she said. "Is there anything you'd like to say?"

Mel looked up from the sand, glancing at each of the faces in the circle. "Devin meant a lot to me, as you all know," she said. The pitch of her voice was suddenly high, and her words almost came out in a squeak. Fresh tears streamed down her face.

"Did you know that he spent time with sick kids?"

Mel nodded toward the sand, and she began to sob uncontrollably. Jenny and Michael wrapped their arms around her, and the rest of the circle followed, closing in on her and surrounding her in a shared embrace.

"I'm so sorry, honey," Donna said.

"Me too," Miriam whispered.

"I'm here for you," Brad said.

"We all are," Haylie offered.

Mel closed her eyes and just stood still. She felt weak for a moment, and as her knees bent ever so slightly, she worried that she might collapse into the sand. But she didn't move an inch.

As everyone else wrapped their arms around her, their strength supported her. And at that moment, she knew it was the only way that she could still be standing on her own two feet.

She was tired.

So incredibly tired of being strong, independent, stubbornly brave and the self-possessed woman that she had been for so long. All of those traits were admirable, she knew, but she had taken them to an extreme. Now was as good a time as any, she figured, to let her friends and her family carry her for a while.

She took a deep breath, and when she let it go, she felt light as a feather.

***

Later that evening, long after the sun had set, Brad started a fire on the beachfront. Spreading blankets and towels on the sand, everyone gathered around and roasted hot dogs and marshmallows, and shared a pack of root beer from Miriam's cooler.

Darius had brought a guitar along and strummed it while Donna beamed proudly, not even flinching when he explained to all that he had learned all of his best songs in prison. Haylie, Jeanette and Jenny chatted about unconventional spellings of baby names, and Miriam made Jenny promise not to give the baby a name like Homer Simpson. Michael and Brad tossed a tennis ball back and forth, playing keep-away, with Bella growing increasingly frustrated in the middle.

And Mel dug her toes in the sand and sat quietly, wondering how their memorial weekend at the beach had suddenly turned into a scene that could have been something painted by Norman Rockwell.

"Hey... I think I'm going to take a walk," Mel said, rising to her feet.

"Want me to come with you?" Jenny offered.

"No thanks," Mel said. "I'll be right back."

Mel walked a parallel path to the shoreline, using the moon and the stars as her compass. After a while, she glanced behind her and realized that she had journeyed much further than she thought she had. The beach house was only a tiny dot of light on the horizon.

She walked toward the barrier of sand dunes separating the houses from the shore, and sank down in a cushion of powdery sand. She closed her eyes and pictured Devin, healed and whole. Without his leg in traction, without a chest tube, without the IV's in his arms and the leads connected to stickers on his chest. Just as he had been before his accident, the handsome and healthy young man that she'd seen on the movie screen dozens of times before.

She pictured him sitting down on the sand next to her. And she remembered the day in the hospital that she took him on an imaginary journey to the ocean.

In her mind, she could hear his voice.

I want us to go together. When I'm well, and I get out of here, I want us to go to the ocean together.

Mel smiled, and her heart seemed to skip a beat.

So it's a date... A day on the beach with the girl I love.

And then Mel wept.

The girl I love. That's who she had been to Devin. Not a rejected woman who had been dumped by her husband; not a financially struggling grandmother-to-be at the age of only forty; not a bitter shrew with a unjustified grudge against the entire male race.

Just the girl he loved.

He had seen in her everything that she could no longer see. Youthfulness, honesty, kindness, her inner beauty and her innate worth. Her right to be valued and cherished – and loved, yes loved – again.

"Oh Devin," she said softly. "I'm so sorry," she wept. "I'm sorry for the pain you felt, and for the way you died, and for the fact that I wasn't there and I couldn't save you. Can you forgive me?"

Mel drew her knees to her chest, wrapped her arms around them, and slowly rocked back and forth in the sand. "Devin," she wept. "I just don't want to say goodbye to you. But I have to."

She took a deep breath and cried for another long while.

"There are still just a few things I need to tell you first," she said.

And in a voice that was little more than a whisper, she spoke softly to Devin and told him how, in a little less than a week, he had completely changed her life.

She told him how he had taught her about forgiveness. In spite of her harsh words and stubborn refusal to be kind to him, he had graciously forgiven her again and again. With each insult, he had turned the other cheek, and had asked for smiles instead of apologies. And it was only because of him that she had found that she could forgive Bruce.

She told him how he had shown her that heroism is not who a person is, but what a person does. And that a person doesn't have to perform showy acts of bravery to be a hero, but that heroism can be found in everyday, humble acts of kindness, compassion and sacrifice. And that people could be heroes to anyone and everyone – from total strangers to close friends and family.

She told him how he had reminded her that children are a blessing, and how it helped her to realize that becoming a grandmother wasn't something to be afraid of.

She told him how she learned from him that life doesn't always unfold according to one's own master plan, but that it could still be a lovely journey. And that joyful experiences were possible even during painful times, and that family and friendship were two threads of comfortable consistency in an ever-changing world.

And that regardless of what had happened in the past, every day could be a new beginning.

She told him that he was the reason that she was ready to love again, and ready to be loved again.

She thanked him, again and again and again.

Then she rose from the sand and pulled a vial of ashes from her pocket. She waded into the water and scattered his heart across the waves.

And when Mel was finally ready, she said goodbye to Devin Ryan, and journeyed back to the beach house to join her friends and family.

Chapter 18
Sunday

During the long ride home on Sunday morning, most of the passengers in Donna's minivan slept, still tired from the late night on the beach.

But Mel was wide awake, still deep in thought; her mind furiously working to process the events of the past two weeks. Her heart was conflicted. Never before had she felt such sadness and a sense of loss, and at the same time, a tremendous feeling of peace and closure.

After a few hours on the road, Mel had exhausted herself in self-reflection and was in desperate need of a distraction. Conversation was out of the question as everyone around her was snoring, except for Donna in the driver's seat. Mel didn't feel like talking to the back of Donna's head and didn't think that her voice could overpower the radio and the blowing air conditioner, anyway.

She reached into her purse, looking for something else to pass the time, and found Friday's mail that she had picked up on the way out the door. Thumbing through it, she didn't see anything very exciting at first. *Power bill, postcard from Michael's optometrist, Chinese food menu, phone bill, letter from Beverly Ryan, pre-approved credit card offer, credit card bill—*

Mel stopped and flipped back to Beverly's letter. She tossed the rest of the mail back into her bag and opened Beverly's note.

My dearest Mel,

I am writing to thank you again for the compassion and kindness that you and your family extended to both myself and my son. I mean it when I say that I don't know how I would have been able to survive his loss without you.

There are some mornings when I wake up and I still can't believe that Devin is gone. And that's just about the time that I turn on the television and see him on the screen in a movie or a news show. I see him in the tabloid racks at the grocery store. I hear his voice on the radio when they replay movie clips and interviews. In an odd little way, the entertainment industry seems to have immortalized my son and if I ever want to see his face or hear his voice, I know he's not that far away. I guess that I'm in a privileged position to be the mother of a movie star, and while the rest of the world mourns him, they're oddly enough keeping him alive for me. Still, Mel, I miss him so. And I know that you do too.

In a small private ceremony today, with my brother and sister and their children, we laid Devin's body to rest, next to his father. Since my husband and son could not be together in life, I have found peace in knowing that they are resting together at last. Their bodies are, anyway. The rest of them, I know, is alive and well, and I carry them both in my spirit.

The next challenging task that I have had to undertake as the administrator of Devin's estate is to decide what to do with his money. As you may have heard, he left a considerable amount of wealth behind. (Oh Mel, why do young people think that they are invincible and never write a will? If only Devin had, he would have spared me a great deal of work!)

I have made some decisions about what to do with his money and I wanted to share these with you. As you and I both know, Devin loved children dearly, and it has guided the choices that I have made in the absence of having a written will. Devin's cousins are all parents with young children. I have set up a trust fund for each child, as I know that Devin would have wanted to give them all a financial foundation for their future. I believe that he would have been content in knowing that they and their families will be able to live comfortably for the rest of their lives.

I have also made contributions to all of the charities that I know of that grant wishes to terminally ill children, as I know that this was another passion of Devin's, and I feel that he would have been happy in this decision.

I have chosen to give the rest of Devin's money to Dogwood Regional Medical Center, to fund the building of the children's hospital. They want to name it the 'Devin Ryan Memorial Children's Hospital at Dogwood.' That has a nice ring to it, doesn't it, Mel? I think I would like that. I want people to remember my son, and this means more to me than all of his movies, awards, and every other praise and accolade that he received as an entertainer.

One more thing, Mel...

In one of our conversations, you told me how Devin had amazed and surprised you during the time that he was hospitalized. You said that in spite of his pain and immobilization, he still managed to laugh and smile and stay in good spirits every day. You told me how Devin showed you that happiness truly is a choice. I think we have lots of choices in life that we don't even realize we have. Like family. We can choose who we want to love and call our family. Devin was the last of my immediate family, but as I told you back in Dogwood, I feel like you are my family now. He loved both of us, and I feel like that has left us with a connection. I am here for you, Mel, just like you were there for me. We can grieve his loss together, and heal together.

I failed to mention earlier that there was one more thing that I chose to do with Devin's estate. Since we are family now, I hope that you will allow Jenny to accept the enclosed gift.

Mel paused and put the letter down. Looking back in the envelope, she found an additional piece of tri-folded paper and unwrapped it. Inside was a smaller piece of paper. Holding it up in front of her eyes to read the small print, she saw that it was a certified bank check, made out to Jennifer Page, in the amount of one million dollars. Mel felt dizzy for a second. She put the check down and took a few deep breaths. Then she resumed reading Beverly's letter.

I think that it will be more than enough to help her get on her feet as a young mother and provide for her baby when it arrives. She's going to be a wonderful mom, and you're going to be a wonderful grandma, Mel. I hope that this gift will take all of the stress and worry out of the baby coming into your lives and allow you to embrace the experience for what it is and what it should be – a blessing, a new adventure in life, and a joy unlike any you've ever known before.

Thank you again for everything, Mel. All of my love to you, Michael, Jenny, and the baby.

Sincerely,
Beverly

Chapter 19
Monday

Every bed on Med-Surg South, except for one, was full. Half of the patients had been admitted during the weekend, and the morning found the nurses so busy that no one had a chance to take a real break. After Mel discharged a patient around noontime, her stomach growled and reminded her that lunch was waiting in the break room fridge. She looked around for Brad, hoping that he could steal a few moments and share a sandwich with her. He was nowhere to be found.

Then she looked for Haylie, thinking that she could chat with her about her new apartment and find out how life in Dogwood Park suited her. Unfortunately she was missing too.

Then she looked for Miriam, knowing that she'd have to endure another several dozen pictures of baby Timothy, with all of his cute facial expressions, ranging from gummy smiles to angry grimaces to looks of drooling indifference. But where was Miriam?

And Donna was nowhere in sight either.

Surely one of them would be hiding out in the break room, taking a moment to catch his or her breath. Mel opened the door, surprised to find that the light was off. She reached to the right and found the switchplate on the wall, flicking the lights on with her index finger.

"Surprise!" Everyone shouted in unison.

Startled, Mel jumped slightly and cupped her hand over her mouth.

Jenny and Michael met her at the door and wrapped their arms around her, pulling her into the break room. "Happy Birthday, Mom!" They giggled.

Donna, Miriam, Brad, and Haylie lined the walls of the tiny room, each holding a wrapped present. "Happy Birthday!" they said again, placing their gifts down on the table and giving Mel a round of applause.

And in the middle of all of them, at the opposite end of the table, was Rodney. He was holding a cake with white frosting and a single lit candle on top of it that looked like a carrot.

"Don't worry," he assured her. "I found a vegetarian birthday cake recipe on the Internet and I tested it out a couple of times before I made this one for you. No eggs, no dairy, no animal products at all. It took some work, but believe it or not, I think I've got it perfected!"

Mel felt her eyes well with tears as she looked around the room at her family and friends. "Oh no," she said, "Here I go, crying again. I guess I should buy stock in the tissue company. Lately I've been their best customer!"

Jenny laughed and shucked a tissue from the dispenser on the wall, passing it to Mel. "Hopefully, you're crying for a happier reason this time," she said, winking at her mother.

"I sure am," Mel laughed. "Thank you all, this means more to me than you'll ever know."

Rodney crossed the room and opened his arms. She stepped toward him and rested her head on his chest as he hugged her. She was delighted to find that he smelled much more like aftershave this time, and a lot less like chicken.

"Just one candle?" She asked.

"Just one," he said with a smile. "To light the way for a new year. And new beginnings that it brings."

Mel sighed contentedly. "I can't thank you enough, Rodney, for being such a good friend. You've been nothing but wonderful since the day I met you. Things have been absolutely crazy for me lately, and they'll probably get even crazier. But please, please don't give up on me. I want you to be a part of my life."

"And I want that, too." He kissed her on the cheek. "So crazy or not, count me in."

She smiled and squeezed him even tighter.

"Happy Birthday, Imelda," he whispered in her ear. "Everything is going to be okay."

"Yes, it is," she agreed.

And for once, she didn't have to believe.

She just knew.

SUGGESTED READING LIST

Although this story about coping with change and loss in nursing is a work of fiction, you can find factual, evidence-based information in professional nursing journals and other published sources. Here are a few suggested resources to enhance your understanding of the concepts depicted in this novella:

Kübler-Ross, Elisabeth. *Living With Death and Dying*. New York: Touchstone, 1997.

Kübler-Ross, Elisabeth. *On Death and Dying*. New York: Touchstone, 1997.
(Additional information and titles by this author may be found at www.elisabethkublerross.com)

Onstott, Anne T. "Perioperative nursing care when sudden patient death occurs in the OR - operating room". <u>AORN Journal</u>. April 1998.

Kurz, Jane M. and Hayes, Evelyn R. (2006) "End of Life Issues Action: Impact of Education," <u>International Journal of Nursing Education Scholarship</u>: Vol. 3 : Iss. 1, Article 18.

Smith-Stoner, Marilyn "Coping with grief and loss." <u>Nursing</u>. February 1998.

O'Lynn, C.E., & Tranbarger, R.E. (Eds.). (2007). <u>Men in nursing: History, challenges and opportunities</u>. New York: Springer.

DISCUSSION GROUP QUESTIONS

1) Which nurse do you relate to the most? Why?

2) Look up Dr. Elisabeth Kübler-Ross's five stages of grief model in your medical library or by Internet search. Can you identify different stages of the model that the individual nurses of Med-Surg South were experiencing?

3) Prior to the deaths of Devin and Amena, each of the nurses had experienced at least one major change in their lives. David explains to the nurses that "all changes are also losses." Do you agree? Why?

4) What has Haylie lost by moving out of her home? What has Donna lost by allowing Darius to move back home? How do they cope?

5) Discuss the nurses' feelings about spirituality. How does it impact their coping skills? How does it impact how they view death and dying?

6) David suggests to the nurses that they need "Spiritual, Emotional and Mental Personal Protective Equipment." Have you personally used any of the ideas that he presented? What else do you do to "protect" yourself from stress, loss and change as a nurse?

7) Have you ever had a patient who was a celebrity or a "V.I.P." like Devin? How did it impact the work environment and patient care?

8) Mel grew attached to Devin, and Brad grew attached to Amena. How were the two attachments different? How were they similar? Did they affect the way that Brad and Mel cared for their patients? Discuss a time that you developed an attachment to a patient and/ or their family.

9) How did the deaths of Devin and Amena impact Mel and Brad?

10) How do nurses typically respond to the death of someone like Amena, an elderly individual who died from an illness? How do nurses typically respond to the death of someone like Devin, a younger individual who died unexpectedly from an injury? Is there a difference? Why or why not?

11) What was different about Amena and Devin's deaths? What is your idea of a "good" death? Who do you think had the better death experience between Amena and Devin?

12) Why do you think that Devin had not yet prepared a will or advanced directives? Do you find that many of your younger adult patients do not have wills and advanced directives?

13) Do you agree with Ms. Ryan's decisions about Devin's remains and the settlement of his estate? Do you think that Devin would have been happy with her decisions?

14) How do Mel and Brad continue to care for Devin and Amena after they have died?

15) Mel and Brad are healers to Devin and Amena. Do you think that Devin and Amena are healers to their nurses in return? Have there ever been times in your nursing career in which your patients were healers for you?

16) Do male nurses deal with the death of a patient differently from female nurses? Why or why not?

17) How was Mel supportive of Beverly after Devin's death?

18) What do you think are the "wrong" things to say to a person who has just lost a loved one? What do you think are the "right" things to say? Or do?

19) Why do you think that the nurses of Med-Surg South held their own memorial ceremony for Amena and Devin?

20) Do you think that Mel decides to let Jenny accept Beverly's gift? Do you think that there are any ethical or moral implications in nurses receiving gifts from patients or their families?

21) How did you see the nurses supporting each other after the losses of the patients? Did you see an instance in which a nurse was not supportive of a fellow nurse grieving a loss?

POST-TEST QUESTIONS

Broken Heart

1) Which of the following statements are true concerning the death of patients?

   a) Nurses should not get attached to patients so that they won't have to mourn the loss if they die

   b) Only loved ones are entitled to grieve the loss of a patient since they have had long-term relationships with those people

   c) A loss of a patient is a loss for a nurse too, and healthy grieving is normal and necessary to be successful as a nurse

   d) a & b

   e) b & c

2) The most appropriate statement to make to a person who has lost a loved one is:

   a) It was his/her time to go

   b) I'm very sorry for your loss

   c) I know exactly how you feel

   d) He/she is in a better place

   e) At least he/she is not suffering anymore

3) What are some things nurses can do to protect themselves spiritually, mentally and emotionally from the demands of their career?

   a) Rest and take breaks

   b) Make contact with a friend

   c) Give advice to others about how to cope

   d) a & b

   e) None of the above

4) Which of the following statements are true about the way nurses grieve?

 a) There is a strong tendency among nurses to deny grief

 b) Male and female nurses tend to grieve exactly the same way

 c) There is a right and a wrong way to grieve

 d) b & c

 e) a & c

5) Which of the nurses was grieving a loss in the story?

 a) Miriam, because her husband had died

 b) Haylie, because she was leaving home and moving away from her mother

 c), Brad, because his girlfriend had left him

 d) Mel and Donna, because there were major changes in the lives of their children

 e) All of the above

6) Which of the following statements are true about the way that nurses cope with loss?

 a) Personal beliefs and faith impact the way that nurses cope

 b) There is a strong tendency among nurses to deny grief

 c) Female nurses tend to express grief more openly and among peers than male nurses do

 d) a & c only

 e) a, b and c

7) Sometimes nurses can hinder the grieving of fellow nurses. An example of this is:

a) Donna asked Mel to consider taking time off or getting help if she was getting overwhelmed by her feelings after Devin's death

b) Miriam took Brad to see the babies to try to teach him something about coping with loss

c) Janice Murphy told Mel to get over Devin's death because she hadn't known him for that long and her grief was creating public relations problems

d) a and c

e) All of the above

8) There is a strong tendency among nurses to deny grief. At what point did a nurse move past denial and begin to grieve?

a) When Haylie went home to talk to her mother

b) When Brad cried in the presence of Miriam, and then privately in his car

c) When Mel went to a private place on the beach to say goodbye to Devin, and then scattered his ashes

d) None of the above; the nurses are all still in denial

e) a, b, and c are all examples of the nurses beginning to accept and grieve their losses

9) Some of the supports and strategies that the nurses used in this story for coping with their losses included:

a) Pastoral care

b) Prayer and Hope

c) Other people – their families, friends, and each other

d) A weekend vacation

e) All of the above

10) Which of the following statements are true?

a) It is common for nurses to place blame when there is a death in the hospital, like the way that Brad blamed Dr. Baylor

b) Whatever cannot be measured in numbers is not considered real in the health care environment and should not be acknowledged

c) When people who have lost a loved one believe that they are experiencing the presence of their deceased friend or family member, it is often just the imagination at work

d) Prayer and meditation can only benefit people who consider themselves religious or spiritual

e) None of the above

CONTINUING NURSING EDUCATION TEST

Broken Heart

Instructions:

- After reading the novella, complete the post-test, the evaluation, and the registration form.

- Mail the completed documents with fee made payable to:
    Department of Nursing Continuing Education
    Southern Regional AHEC
    1601 Owen Drive
    Fayetteville, NC 28304

- Within 4-6 weeks after we receive your paperwork and with successful completion of the post-test, your continuing education certificate will be mailed to you. Passing score is 80%. If you fail, you have the option of retaking the test at no additional cost

- Questions? Contact SRAHEC Department of Nursing Continuing Education at 910-678-7216 or 910-678-7246.

Provider Accreditation (readers are eligible for 3.5 contact hours, CNE)

Southern Regional AHEC is approved as a provider of continuing nursing education by the North Carolina Nurses Association, an accredited approver by the American Nurses Credentialing Center's Commission on Accreditation.

AP#005-607

Payment

The registration fee for this test is $10.00 per person. Checks should be made payable to "Southern Regional AHEC". We also accept Visa and MasterCard. Do not send cash with your paperwork. Institutional/bulk discounts for ten or more tests are available. Please call 910-678-7216 for more information.

Purpose of this educational activity:

Broken Heart is an educational fiction novella (short novel) about coping with change and loss. Through a fiction story, readers will follow a cast of 5 nursing characters at a hospital's Med-Surg unit. Brad and Mel, the two main characters in the story, become attached to patients who die. Each of the other nurses are coping with a major loss or life change of some kind, so the team pulls together and supports each other throughout the difficult time. The hospital chaplain provides advice and information on coping with change and loss, and the nurses explore grieving as a group, and individually. The story helps the reader identify the nurse's need to grieve loss, learn tips for coping with stress caused by loss, and review the different ways that nurses grieve.

Learning Objectives:

Upon completion of this educational activity, the participant should be able to:

1) Explain why every change is also a loss

2) Discuss the nurse's need to grieve the loss of a patient

3) Discuss how grieving behaviors differ between male and female nurses

4) Describe how nurses can support the patient, the family and loved ones, and each other when preparing for or recovering from a patient's death

CNE ENROLLMENT FORM

Broken Heart

CASCE # 27317

Please print or type. All fields must be completed in order to score the test and award continuing education credits. Incomplete enrollment forms will be returned.

Name _____

❑ RN ❑ LPN ❑ NP ❑ CRNA ❑ Student ❑ Other _____

Address _____

Last 4 digits of SSN: XXX-XX-_____

City _____

State _____ Zip Code _____

Home Phone _____

Email _____

Employer _____

Job Title _____

Work Address _____

Area of Specialty _____

Work City _____

State _____ Zip Code _____

Work Phone _____

Work Email _____

Amount enclosed $10.00 paid by:

❏ Check enclosed (made payable to "SRAHEC")   ❏ MasterCard   ❏ Visa

Credit card # _____

Expiration date _____

Signature _____

Last 3 digits on signature panel _____

TEST ANSWERS

Place an "X" through your answer to each question

1. A	B	C	D
2. A	B	C	D
3. A	B	C	D
4. A	B	C	D
5. A	B	C	D
6. A	B	C	D
7. A	B	C	D
8. A	B	C	D
9. A	B	C	D
10. A	B	C	D

ACTIVITY EVALUATION

1. The course content was pertinent to my educational needs and practice

❏ Strongly Agree   ❏ Agree   ❏ Neutral   ❏ Disagree   Strongly
                       ❏ N/A   ❏ Disagree

2. Course objectives were met

❏ Strongly Agree   ❏ Agree   ❏ Neutral   ❏ Disagree   Strongly
                       ❏ N/A   ❏ Disagree

3. I will be able to incorporate what I learned into my practice

❏ Strongly Agree   ❏ Agree   ❏ Neutral   ❏ Disagree   Strongly
                       ❏ N/A   ❏ Disagree

Comments: _____

_____

_____

_____

_____

_____

Mail this form with your payment to:

         Department of Nursing Continuing Education
         Southern Regional AHEC
         1601 Owen Drive
         Fayetteville, NC 28304

www.ingramcontent.com/pod-product-compliance
Lightning Source LLC
Chambersburg PA
CBHW071253220526
45468CB00001B/110